PARAMEDIC REVIEW GUIDE

Brady

PARAMEDIC REVIEW GUIDE

Case Studies and Self-Assessment Questions

Gail Walraven

Miles Julihn

BRADY
PRENTICE HALL
Englewood Cliffs, New Jersey 07632

Library of Congress Cataloging-in-Publication Data

Walraven, Gail, 1949–
Paramedic review guide.

"A Brady book."
Rev. ed. of: Paramedic field review. c1982.
Includes index.
1. Medical emergencies—Case studies. 2. Medical emergencies—Examinations, questions, etc. I. Julihn, Miles. II. Walraven, Gail, 1949– . Paramedic field review. III. Title. [DNLM: 1. Emergency Medicine —case studies. 2. Emergency Medicine—examination questions. WB 18 W221p]
RC86.7.W358 1987 616'.025'076 88-2488
ISBN 0-89303-751-6

Editorial/production supervision
and interior design: *Anne Kenney*
Cover design: *Lundgren Graphics, Ltd.*
Manufacturing buyer: *Peter Havens*

Previously published as PARAMEDIC FIELD REVIEW Case Studies and Self-Assessment Questions, Walraven and Julihn, Reston, 1982.

The care procedures presented here represent accepted practices in the United States. They are not offered as a standard of care. EMT-Advanced emergency care is to be performed under the authority and guidance of a licensed physician. It is the reader's responsibility to know and follow local care protocols as provided by the medical advisors directing the system to which he or she belongs. Also, it is the reader's responsibility to stay informed of emergency care procedure changes.

Printed in the United States of America

10 9 8 7 6 5

ISBN 0-89303-751-6

Prentice-Hall International (UK) Limited, *London*
Prentice-Hall of Australia Pty. Limited, *Sydney*
Prentice-Hall Canada Inc., *Toronto*
Prentice-Hall Hispanoamericana, S.A., *Mexico*
Prentice-Hall of India Private Limited, *New Delhi*
Prentice-Hall of Japan, Inc., *Tokyo*
Simon & Schuster Asia Pte. Ltd., *Singapore*
Editora Prentice-Hall do Brasil, Ltda., *Rio de Janeiro*

CONTENTS

PREFACE

In this book the reader will find a resource of challenging self-assessment exercises corresponding to the fifteen modules of the current National Highway Traffic Safety Administration's national paramedic curriculum. Each chapter contains prehospital case studies, which ask for reader interaction to manage the patient. The case studies are followed by multiple-choice self-assessment questions related to the topics contained in each module. While not designed to review thoroughly every topic in the national curriculum, the book does contain 41 case studies and approximately 640 self-assessment questions.

Many case studies and the self-assessment questions came from the authors' previously published monthly features in *Emergency: The Journal of Emergency Services,* which have enjoyed a wide readership. It is hoped that this book will be helpful to students and certified paramedics alike for keeping their knowledge current, as well as provide an aid in preparing for certification exams.

In both the case studies and the self-assessment questions, the reader is to select the single best answer. Although every effort has been made to avoid ambiguity, some controversies may arise, based upon local protocols and training. In all areas relating to advanced cardiac life support, the authors have adhered to the most recent standards sanctioned by the American Heart Association and published in the *Journal of the American Medical Association* (*JAMA,* June 1986). All electrocardiographs included in the text should be interpreted as a standard lead II configuration. The reader should also keep in mind that EKG strips have been selected for conditions realistically encountered in the field and to identify the basic underlying rhythm. The patient is to be treated only in cases of a symptomatic arrhythmia.

It is hoped that as you are challenged by this book, it will be translated into patient care that is caring, competent, and rewarding.

GAIL WALRAVEN
MILES JULIHN

Editor's Note:
This text was formerly published by Reston Publishing Company, Inc. under the title *Paramedic Field Review.* Brady revised this text with a new title and its logo because of the quality of the material and authors. Six new case studies have been added and the Advanced Cardiac Life Support material has been updated. We are pleased to add this text to our EMS product line.

1

THE EMT-P: ROLE AND LEGAL RESPONSIBILITY

CASE STUDY 1A: THE STUDENT PARAMEDIC

You arrive at the firehouse at your customary time, 7:30 A.M. That leaves you 30 minutes to change into your uniform, grab a cup of coffee, and scan the morning newspaper before the start of your 24-hour shift at 8:00. This morning, however, you are expecting a temporary addition to the paramedic crew, a new student paramedic. You and your partner have trained many and take pride in the fact that all but one have been able to meet your rigorous requirements leading to certification.

"Hi, I'm one of your paramedic evaluators," you say with a friendly, outstretched hand as you sit down at the kitchen table. "You must be our new student."

"Yes, I am. I've heard a lot of good things about the program here, so I'm glad that they assigned me to this station."

"This is my partner, your other evaluator during your 20 or so shifts with us," you say as your partner sits down, coffee cup in hand.

The paramedic instructors from the medical school's teaching hospital have told you little about your new intern, other than that the intern has been a very good student and has some experience working for a private ambulance company. Your job is to observe and evaluate the intern's knowledge, skills, attitude, and performance under stress along with a dozen or more other factors that will ultimately determine the competence to be certified.

You begin: "The first thing we want you to do this morning, is just familiarize yourself with the paramedic unit. Find out where everything is kept and don't be afraid to ask questions."

"Great. I'll get started now," your student says enthusiastically.

"Oh, by the way, we will handle the first call today while you observe," your partner points out. "After that, you'll be the patient medic, so be ready."

"Sounds fine to me." With that the intern goes to the apparatus floor.

Over the next few shifts you and your partner work closely with the new student. Oral quizzes on drug dosages, indications, and contraindications are given informally on a daily basis. Together you determine his knowledge of airway management, priorities in multiple trauma, legal issues, cardiac arrhythmias, and other vital areas.

On his third shift you are observing your student as he deals with a victim of obvious alcohol intoxication. The belligerent patient refuses to be treated and tells the intern to leave him alone. The intern calmly but firmly insists on performing a brief physical exam even though threatened by the patient.

Which of the following legal considerations should you later discuss with the inexperienced intern:

1. abandonment
2. consent
3. battery
4. tort law

Proper consent is vital to respecting patient rights. While often informal in the prehospital setting consent must be granted by a conscious patient prior to any field evaluation or treatment.

After several more shifts you and your partner are pleased with the depth of the intern's medical knowledge. With some initial coaching his intravenous (IV) technique has improved remarkably. Although his assessment skills are adequate, he seems unable to establish rapport and instill confidence in patients.

Which of these would be the least helpful to the intern in developing rapport with patients:

1. Identifying himself (herself) initially and reassuring the patient.
2. Using phrases like "I'll bet it only hurts when you laugh," etc.
3. Briefly explaining procedures to be performed to the patient (IVs, nasal oxygen, etc.).
4. Asking the patient's name and using it frequently.

Encouraging a patient's confidence and trust is an invaluable skill. Often the patient may be very anxious, fearful about what is wrong and what is going to happen. Use of cliches and attempts at humor are often inappropriate and unprofessional as well. Being honest and optimistic is more likely to reassure the patient and put him or her at ease.

On the morning of his tenth shift, your intern is assigned as radio medic for the day. He has operated the paramedic radio properly thus far but has not yet experienced a stressful call in this role. At 9:30 A.M. your unit responds to a parachute accident at a recreational area just outside town. The patient is unconscious upon your arrival. Witnesses report that the patient's chute failed to open fully. There are obvious head and chest injuries as well as multiple fractures. Immediate stabilization and transport are indicated for this critical patient. Upon his initial contact with the hospital, the flustered intern gives such a jumbled and sketchy radio report that time is needlessly wasted and treatment delayed.

Realizing his failure to perform well under stress, the intern sheepishly asks for your comments on the ride back from the hospital.

In your response you should probably refrain from

1. clearly expressing your personal disappointment
2. identifying specific problem areas
3. defining exactly what should have been done
4. reinforcing positive aspects of his performance

While performance under stressful circumstances is an extremely important skill to master, failure in this and other areas can be used as a learning experience. Expressing your personal disappointment is generally not helpful. Instead, criticism can be constructive and should encourage the learner to achieve defined behavioral objectives.

On the following shift your paramedic unit is assigned a public relations talk for a local businessmen's luncheon. While not always convenient and often repetitive, educating the public is an important part of your job. This time you've asked the intern to speak to the group. You and your partner thoroughly discuss the topic with him prior to the meeting. Then your partner reminds him to shine his boots before you go, to emphasize the importance of his professional appearance.

An appropriate topic for a presentation to this typical adult audience might be

1. the value of citizen CPR
2. access to emergency medical services
3. accidental poisoning in children
4. any of the above

Any of the given topics could be addressed. You and your partner select "access to emergency medical services" and remind the intern to include information about available paramedic service, emergency phone numbers, information needed by the dispatcher from the caller, first responders, and typical medical emergencies handled by paramedics.

It is the intern's final shift with you and your partner. He has mastered his clinical skills rapidly, and his knowledge of pharmacology, cardiac arrhythmias, treatment protocols, and medical management are above average. He has responded eagerly to criticism and has displayed the highest degree of professional ethics and behavior. You and your partner are able to recommend his certification strongly.

RELATED ASSESSMENT QUESTIONS

1.1 If a patient refuses treatment but you forcibly proceed to give an injection, you are
(a) guilty of libel
(b) committing battery
(c) operating under implied consent
(d) avoiding a charge of negligence
(e) legally protected if you use sound medical judgment

1.2 An ambulance attendant who has been trained under the Department of Transportation curriculum for advanced life support and who is able to administer advanced, invasive treatments such as drugs, IVs, and defibrillation, is qualified for certification as
(a) an EMT-I (non-ambulance)
(b) an EMT-I (ambulance)
(c) an EMT-D
(d) an EMT-paramedic
(e) an EMT-physician's assistant

1.3 Which of the following is responsible for coordinating all emergency medical response and treatment activities within a city, or county, region:
(a) the hospital council
(b) the ambulance association
(c) the local ACEP chapter
(d) the EMS agency
(e) the fire department

1.4 Your patient is a chronic alcoholic who appears intoxicated and is complaining of nausea. The patient seems very stable, but you give oxygen and start a TKO IV as a routine precaution. While preparing to transport, you are told of a full arrest in progress in your district. You quickly call an EMT ambulance to your scene to transport the alcoholic, and you proceed to the full arrrest, without waiting for the EMT's to arrive. This action constitutes
(a) abandonment
(b) legal prioritization
(c) tort infringement
(d) assault
(e) misdemeanor delay

1.5 Your patient is awake and alert following a traffic accident but has major chest and abdominal trauma. You prepare to start an IV, but the patient refuses for religious reasons. You can

(a) go ahead and start the IV since this is an emergency
(b) start the IV because the patient doesn't know what's best for him/her
(c) get a police officer to declare the patient incompetent, then start the IV
(d) wait for the patient to lose consciousness, then start the IV
(e) try to talk the patient into the IV, then start it if he/she gives permission

1.6 In which of the following situations would it be illegal for a paramedic to start an IV:

(a) when directed by a physician at the scene of a disaster
(b) when standing orders apply
(c) when ordered by a mobile intensive care nurse over the radio from the hospital
(d) when ordered by a physician in the emergency department
(e) when communication with the hospital isn't possible, but the patient will die without the IV

1.7 You respond to a child hit by a car. The child is unconscious and bleeding badly. The child's parents are not around. You should

(a) go ahead and treat the child, since this is an emergency
(b) withhold all treatment until parents can give consent
(c) withhold invasive treatment and transport immediately
(d) send a police officer to get parental consent
(e) have the police get a court order over the radio

1.8 You are legally able to treat a patient who is unconscious because

(a) the patient has not refused care
(b) it would be negligent not to treat the patient
(c) the patient's consent is implied
(d) you have an ethical obligation
(e) the Good Samaritan Act protects you

1.9 Your patient is confused, disoriented, and exhibiting bizarre behavior. The patient's son tells you that the patient was recently released from a mental hospital, and now the son wants the patient returned. The patient refuses transport. You can forcibly restrain and transport this patient only if

(a) the son signs a consent
(b) the patient loses consciousness
(c) it has been less than 72 hours since the patient was released
(d) a police officer will attest that the patient is a danger to himself/herself or others
(e) your hospital will agree to the action

1.10 You are unable to defibrillate a patient because the defibrillator doesn't charge. The patient later dies, and the family learns that you failed to replace the battery that morning according to routine procedures. They can sue you for
(a) negligence
(b) malpractice
(c) abandonment
(d) deceit
(e) tort violation

1.11 Which of the following is *not* necessary to prove in order to find a paramedic guilty of negligence:
(a) the paramedic had a duty to act
(b) that the paramedic didn't perform as another prudent paramedic would
(c) that the patient was injured
(d) that the injury was a result of the paramedic's action
(e) that the paramedic was aware that he/she might be causing injury

ANSWER KEY

1.1 b	**1.4** a	**1.7** a	**1.10** a
1.2 d	**1.5** e	**1.8** c	**1.11** e
1.3 d	**1.6** e	**1.9** d	

2

HUMAN SYSTEMS AND PATIENT ASSESSMENT

CASE STUDY 2A: CME CLASS ON PATIENT ASSESSMENT

It is your day off, but you and your partner have planned to attend a presentation on Patient Assessment for Paramedics, sponsored by a local hospital for continuing medical education (CME) credit. You both have worked together for three years since completing paramedic school, and your assessment skills are sharp. Nevertheless, it is hoped that the presentation will enable you to be even more proficient.

As you enter the small auditorium on the ground floor of the hospital, you are given a course outline along with other pertinent materials. Free coffee and doughnuts are available at a table in the rear of the room and you recognize some old faces gathered there. You swap war stories as other members of the prehospital team filter in. Soon the lecture is ready to begin.

The master of ceremonies introduces the chief of internal medicine at the local hospital, who rises, stands behind the podium, and begins: "Good morning. I know that most of you are here not because it's the best thing you can think of to be doing, but because many of you are probably short on CME units this quarter." A chuckle ripples through the audience. "In the packets you received when you came in are several numbered response cards that I will ask you to fill out at various times throughout the program. I hope they will provide a catalyst for discussion.

"As you know, patient assessment actually begins before prehospital responders ever reach the patient. Upon arriving at the scene, it is important to observe the environment and the setting. Often, available clues may be significant in determining what to look for or suspect when we actually examine the patient. If, for example, we arrive at the scene of a vehicle accident and notice a 'starred' windshield, multiple cracks in the laminated glass radiating outward from a single point of impact, we would definitely look for signs of head injury and suspect a possible cervical injury. In addition, if we observed arcing power lines down at the scene, we would take necessary precautions to protect ourselves and any patients from contact with the live wires. Other hazards to rescue personnel and victims should also be considered: spilled fuel, fire, person with a gun, toxic atmospheres, or imminent structural collapse.

"Once we become involved in the scene, it becomes very difficult to see what is going on around us. The need for additional personnel and equipment must also be recognized soon after our arrival. When we roll alone on that infamous 'man down' call and discover a patient in cardiac arrest, we must immediately decide if additional personnel can be obtained in order to perform advanced life support measures in the field. Thus, a lot of information may be available to us if we only will look for it as we approach the scene.

"As we approach the patient, we must have a plan or system for examination. Far from being strict or rigid, our system must be flexible, yet complete. Since some information is more important and must precede others, we will prioritize our assessment and perform the most vital functions first.

"Now if you will, please respond to card 1 from your packet" It reads, The Primary Survey focuses on

1. vital signs
2. ABC's
3. deep tendon reflexes
4. chief complaint

"A good place to start, at least with a conscious patient, is to identify yourself and your role. Thus, you might begin with something like 'Hi, my name is So-and-So and I'm a paramedic with the fire department.' This aids in establishing good rapport and helps an apprehensive patient to be more cooperative.

"Immediately after identifying ourselves, we must assure that there is adequate airway, breathing, and circulation. If the airway is obstructed or breathing is noisy, immediate steps must be taken to establish a patent airway. If breathing is very shallow or absent, then ventilation will be initiated. If the pulse is absent or very slow, CPR may be indicated. Until adequate ventilation and circulation are maintained either spontaneously or artificially, your assessment can go no farther. In a conscious patient who is alert and has no respiratory distress, the airway and breathing are obviously intact. A quick check of the pulse allows you to proceed to the next phase, which is the secondary survey.

"First we need to identify the chief complaint. Often it may be obvious why you were called, but it is always wise to have the patient tell you where he or she hurts, how the patient feels, or what happened. Since pain is one of the most frequent chief complaints encountered by paramedics, here is a helpful mnemonic to remember when evaluating this complaint."

The speaker goes to an overhead projector and displays a slide (Table 2-1).

"You can now respond to card 2."

It reads, Which of these is not an appropriate description of a patient with a decreased level of consciousness:

1. semicomatose
2. alert and oriented
3. responds to deep pain
4. conscious but confused

"What about the patient who is unconscious, has an altered level of consciousness, or is otherwise unable to verbalize his chief complaint? In such cases where there is no obvious chief complaint such as cardiac arrest, head injury, multiple trauma, or overdose, then we must describe the patient's level of consciousness. The use of terms as obtunded, semicomatose, lethargic, stage II coma, etc., should be avoided, because such terminology is ambiguous and often misinterpreted by others.

"Instead, we identify whether the patient is awake (conscious) or not (unconscious). If the patient is awake, we must determine whether the patient is oriented. The patient may be alert, confused, combative, or anywhere in between. The level of orientation is evaluated on the basis of whether the patient knows who he (or she) is (person), where he (or she) is (place), and what time or day it is (time). If the patient can correctly respond to all three, then

TABLE 2–1 Evaluation of the Chief Complaint

P (provokes):	What seemed to bring on the pain? What was the patient doing when it started? (*Note:* It may be unprovoked.)
Q (quality):	Can the patient describe the pain? Is it sharp? dull? a pressure? burning or stabbing?
R (region and radiation):	Where is the pain located anatomically? Does the pain travel anywhere else?
S (severity):	Have the patient rate the pain on a scale of 1 to 10, where 10 is the worst pain he has ever had.
T (time):	When did the pain start? Does it come and go?

the patient is alert and oriented. If the patient is unconscious, we will describe how the patient responds to both verbal and pain stimuli. The important thing to remember is to describe specifically how the patient responds and to what stimulus. Remember also that a patient can be described as both unconscious and unresponsive.''

The speaker moves back to the overhead projector.

''With an unconscious patient, another mnemonic may be helpful. It is called BRIM (Table 2–2).

''Changes in skin color, temperature, and moisture can be early clues to the patient's level of perfusion. In fact, impending shock and accompanying changes in hemodynamic balance can often be more quickly diagnosed by such abnormal findings as pale, cool, and clammy skin than by changes in vital signs. The patient's skin is usually readily accessible and should be evaluated early in the secondary survey.

''Vital signs should also be taken as part of the secondary survey. Pulse would include rate and rhythm (regular or irregular), and it should be noted if it was taken apically by auscultation or peripherally by palpation. Respirations should be reported in terms of rate, rhythm, and quality (deep, labored, shallow). Blood pressure is simply reported as systolic over diastolic. If palpation is used, it should also be noted.

''At this point in your patient assessment you should have the following information: the scene, the patient's sex, estimated age and weight, chief complaint, skin signs, and vital signs. With this information you should be able to classify your patient's overall status into one of the three categories: mild, moderate, or severe.

''Please refer to response card 3.''

It reads, Your patient is a 42-year-old male with substernal chest pain. His electrocardiogram (EKG) shows normal sinus rhythm with multifocal PVC's. His status would be

1. mild
2. moderate
3. severe
4. stable

TABLE 2–2 Evaluation of the Unconscious Patient

B (*b*reathing):	Rate, rhythm, quality, patterns
R (*r*esponse):	How does the patient respond when stimulated by verbal command or pain?
I (*eyes*):	Pupil size, reaction to light, equality
M (*m*ovement):	Does the patient have any spontaneous or directed movement of his extremities? Is he posturing?

"Since triaging patients into a particular category is seldom easy, consider the following guidelines:

- *Mild:* Patients in this category require little or no prehospital care. Generally these conditions are nonemergent in nature: minor lacerations, fractures, flu-like symptoms, elevated temperature, postseizure, etc.
- *Moderate:* Patients in this category have the potential to deteriorate, and drug therapy may be required. It would include arrhythmias, seizures, altered level of consciousness, femoral fractures, and most burns. Incidentally, your patient with chest pain would be placed in this category.
- *Severe:* Patients who are severe require immediate advanced life support in the field and prompt transport. This category would include multiple trauma, respiratory distress, cardiac arrest, uncontrolled hemorrhage, life-threatening arrhythmias, and severe head injury.

"Of course, at any point in our primary or secondary survey when treatment is deemed necessary (i.e., oxygen, suctioning, CPR, control bleeding, extrication, cardiac monitoring, etc.), it is initiated without delay.

"Take a look at card 4."

It reads, Which of the following is *least* important when obtaining the patient's medical history:

1. current or recent illnesses
2. prescribed medications
3. drug allergies
4. immunizations

"During the course of your patient assessment, it is important to ask pertinent questions regarding the patient's current or recent illnesses, prescribed medications, and allergies to drugs. A history of immunizations is generally not relevant. Special questions may be appropriate, especially when exploring the chief complaint. This information can be very helpful in providing the hospital a complete picture of your patient's medical emergency.

"Of course, your secondary survey is not complete until you perform a thorough physical exam. Following a head-to-toe approach, we will examine the patient further for significant findings that will aid in establishing a working diagnosis and determining an appropriate course of treatment.

"Starting with the head, we will look for any obvious injury to this vital area. Lacerations are usually very apparent owing to profuse bleeding; however, they can be difficult to locate, especially in the hair. Feel for deformity and depressions that might indicate damage to the skull itself. Check ear canals for bleeding or traces of cerebrospinal fluid. If you have not already done so, examine pupils for size, equality, and reaction to light. Note any particular odor on the breath that might be indicative of alcohol intoxication, ketoacidosis, etc. Have the patient clinch his/her teeth together to see if they meet normally. Palpate the face gently for areas of tenderness. In the neck we will check for tenderness to palpation especially the cervical spine, and note any deformity. In a nontrauma patient the neck may be flexed to check for any nuchal rigidity. Neck veins should be checked for distention, and pulse may be palpated at the carotid arteries. The trachea should be in the midline.

"The chest will be examined by observation, palpation, auscultation, and, rarely, percussion. The anterior chest wall should be observed for equal bilateral expansion with each respiratory effort. Any retraction at the sternal notch, between the ribs, or below the costal margin should be noted. Obvious trauma to the chest, including the back, should also be checked. Palpation will reveal any crepitus or areas of tenderness. Auscultation of breath sounds should be performed bilaterally in both upper and lower lobes. In addition, heart sounds can be auscultated for valvular insufficiency (if you are really good) and apical pulse. Percussion is only of limited value in the field in cases of suspected pneumothorax. The spine should be palpated for areas of tenderness and possible deformity. A knowledge of key anatomic landmarks will be helpful in identifying injuries along the spine as well as the chest.

"The abdomen, too, is inspected for any signs of trauma such as lacerations, gunshot wound, eviscerated organs, or ecchymosis. In addition, the abdomen is palpated in all four quadrants for tenderness, guarding, masses, and rigidity. Bowel sounds may be auscultated; keep in mind that a minimum of 30 to 60 seconds is necessary to suspect that bowel sounds are absent. The pelvis is stressed by compression on the iliac crests bilaterally and the symphysis pubis anteriorly for any pain response that might be elicited.

"Each arm and leg should be examined for possible injury, especially swelling, deformity, and tenderness. If no significant injury is visible, the limb should be moved voluntarily by the patient through a full range of motion. It should also be determined if there is any loss of sensation. In addition, have the patient squeeze your index fingers simultaneously with his or her hands to see if grip strengths are equal. Finally, have the patient dorsiflex and plantarflex each foot against some resistance.

"Let me leave you with this parting thought," concludes the lecturer. "No other skill learned by the EMT-paramedic has perhaps more influence on effective delivery of prehospital care than the ability to evaluate patients accurately and rapidly in the field. The ability to observe, interpret, and communicate meaningful data comes easily only to some and naturally to none. This skill is mastered through experience and a systematic approach time after time. Ultimately, a patient's outcome may well depend upon your accurate assessment of his medical emergency."

The two-hour session has passed very quickly. You and your partner are left with some new tools and valuable insights that will make the job that you do that much better.

RELATED ASSESSMENT QUESTIONS

2.1 Which of the following would be the *least* appropriate field use for auscultation:

(a) determining heart rate
(b) listening for breath sounds
(c) detecting "muffled" heart sounds
(d) auscultating bowel sounds
(e) checking proper placement of an endotracheal tube

2.2 While auscultating an apical heart beat, it is often helpful to have the patient

(a) cough
(b) hold his or her breath
(c) do a Valsalva maneuver
(d) hyperventilate
(e) describe his complaint

2.3 Auscultation of breath sounds is an important aspect of all of the following procedures except

(a) insertion of an EOA
(b) administration of IV fluids
(c) cannulation of the subclavian vein
(d) application of antishock trousers
(e) venipuncture to obtain a blood sample

2.4 Hypertension is usually considered to begin when the diastolic blood pressure exceeds

(a) 80
(b) 90
(c) 100
(d) 110
(e) 120

2.5 Hypotension is defined as

(a) systolic BP less than 100
(b) diastolic BP less than 60
(c) BP lower than usual for that patient
(d) BP lower than average for the patient's age group
(e) BP with less than 20 points between the systolic and diastolic

2.6 A "normal" blood pressure for a 20-year-old male is

(a) 100/60
(b) 110/80
(c) 130/90
(d) 120/80
(e) 150/100

2.7 A "normal" pulse range for an adult is
(a) 60–100
(b) 75–110
(c) 50–80
(d) 65–85
(e) 80–120

2.8 A "normal" adult respiratory rate is
(a) 16–20
(b) 8–16
(c) 20–28
(d) 24–30
(e) 8–12

Medical Terminology Exercise

Directions: Match the terms in column A with the closest definition in column B

Column A		Column B
2.9	dys-	a. see, visualize
2.10	neuro-	b. eye
2.11	c̄	c. muscle
2.12	s̄	d. painful, bad
2.13	p̄	e. blood
2.14	anti-	f. against
2.15	myo-	g. surgical removal
2.16	-ology	h. double
2.17	-ostomy	i. fast
2.18	bolus	j. in one mass
2.19	hemo-	k. bone
2.20	-itis	l. nerves
2.21	pneu-	m. head
2.22	tachy-	n. within
2.23	osteo-	o. inflammation
2.24	hyper-	p. heart
2.25	antero-	q. with
2.26	optho-	r. make an opening
2.27	-ectomy	s. air, lungs
2.28	hematoma	t. without
2.29	intra-	u. bruise
2.30	cardio-	v. in front
2.31	cephalo-	w. study
2.32	diplo-	x. after
2.33	-scopy	y. above

Anatomy and Physiology Exercise

Directions: Match the terms in column A with the closest definition in Column B

Column A	Column B
2.34 CNS	a. kidneys, ureters, bladder, and urethra
2.35 colon	b. upper chambers of the heart
2.36 phalanges	c. main artery leading from the heart
2.37 atria (auricles)	d. large intestine
2.38 aorta	e. brain, brain stem, and spinal cord
2.39 pancreas	f. main vessel returning blood from the lower part of the body to the heart
2.40 excretory system	g. organ that stores bile
2.41 alveoli	h. skull bone
2.42 larynx	i. secretes epinephrine
2.43 esophagus	j. nervous system consisting of sympathetic and parasympathetic branches
2.44 gall bladder	k. bones of the hip girdle
2.45 sternum	l. voice box
2.46 pelvis	m. bones of the spinal column
2.47 vertebrae	n. knee cap
2.48 inferior vena cava	o. site of oxygen exchange in the tissues
2.49 autonomic nervous system	p. bones of the fingers and toes
2.50 capillaries	q. gland that produces insulin
2.51 cranium	r. passage between the mouth and stomach
2.52 adrenal glands	s. terminal air sacs in lungs
2.53 patella	t. breastbone

ANSWER KEY

2.1 d	**2.14** f	**2.27** g	**2.40** a
2.2 b	**2.15** c	**2.28** u	**2.41** s
2.3 e	**2.16** w	**2.29** n	**2.42** l
2.4 b	**2.17** r	**2.30** p	**2.43** r
2.5 c	**2.18** j	**2.31** m	**2.44** g
2.6 d	**2.19** e	**2.32** h	**2.45** t
2.7 a	**2.20** o	**2.33** a	**2.46** k
2.8 a	**2.21** s	**2.34** e	**2.47** m
2.9 d	**2.22** i	**2.35** d	**2.48** f
2.10 l	**2.23** k	**2.36** p	**2.49** j
2.11 q	**2.24** y	**2.37** b	**2.50** o
2.12 t	**2.25** v	**2.38** c	**2.51** h
2.13 x	**2.26** b	**2.39** q	**2.52** i
			2.53 n

3

SHOCK AND FLUID THERAPY

CASE STUDY 3A: MR. E. LUTHER

You are notified by the highway patrol to respond to a vehicle accident. No further details are given. Your normal response is one paramedic ambulance with two medics aboard and one engine company with four people. Upon arrival you find that two automobiles have collided head on. There is severe damage to both vehicles; a highway patrol officer tells you that six victims are involved. As radio medic, you are designated the triage officer. What would you do first:

1. set up traffic control to protect the scene
2. triage all patients to ascertain the extent of injuries
3. request additional equipment and personnel
4. establish radio communication with the hospital

All of the above are important, and each must be considered in short order by the paramedic team. Because there are six victims to assess, however, additional support in personnel and equipment is probably required.

After examination of the victims, you find that one is pulseless and apneic, one has a critical chest injury and is trapped in the car, one has a severe head injury, and the remaining three have minor injuries. A second ambulance has arrived. Which patient(s) do you treat first:

1. victim who is pulseless and apneic
2. victim with head injury
3. victim with chest injury
4. victims with minor injuries

The basic principle to follow in triage of a multipatient incident is to do the most good for the most people. A pulseless, apneic victim is considered a low priority unless sufficient personnel is available. The best way to set priorities is to follow the ABCs. Any significant chest injury is likely to interfere with the airway and respiratory efforts; thus, this patient is your first concern. You assign your partner to assess the patient.

Your next priority is the patient with a head injury. Any victim with a severe head injury also demands immediate attention. A patient who is unconscious with severe head trauma requires immediate transport. You decide to transport this patient via EMT ambulance. The patient's neck is immobilized and is placed on a backboard. Which of the following is the most important instruction to give to the competent EMT attendant:

1. maintain the airway and hyperventilate with O_2
2. repeat vital signs every three minutes
3. keep the patient supine, head turned to the side
4. check frequently for unequal pupils

In these choices nothing is as important to stress as an adequate airway and high flow oxygen. Signs of an extending head injury (i.e., deteriorating vital signs, posturing, unequal pupils, etc.) are important to observe if conditions permit. However, little other treatment can be initiated in the prehospital phase.

You find your partner, who is inside one of the demolished vehicles with the chest injury patient. Engine company personnel are performing extrication. The patient is a 30-year-old male who is conscious but confused. There is obvious blunt trauma to the chest with paradoxical respirations, and he is complaining of severe chest pain. The abdomen is markedly tender in the right upper quadrant. Vital signs are pulse 140, respirations 32 and labored, B/P 106/88. Radio contact with the hospital is attempted but there is no response. Which of these actions would you take first:

1. inform the officer in charge
2. quickly troubleshoot your communications system
3. complete extrication and transport stat
4. relay information to the hospital via your dispatcher

Communication is the vital link in most systems for initiating paramedic level treatment in the field. When communication cannot be established by normal means, alternatives must be considered. But, in every case, be sure to recheck your equipment for the obvious: wrong channel, antenna not hooked up, low battery, etc. In this case, replacing the weak battery brings in the hospital loud and clear.

The order that you would least expect to receive after giving your initial assessment is

1. IV Ringer's lactate
2. morphine sulfate (MS), up to 6 mg IV
3. monitor the EKG
4. O_2 at 6 to 8 LPM

Morphine sulfate is the only suggested order contraindicated for this patient. This drug is a potent CNS depressant and can mask symptoms in a patient with multisystem trauma. In addition, MS is also a vasodilator that could be lethal to this shocky patient.

The patient is finally removed from the wreckage, but his level of consciousness is decreasing. Your partner gives you new vital signs: pulse 140, respirations 36 and shallow, B/P 70/50. Breath sounds appear to be slightly diminished on the right side. Two IVs of Ringer's lactate have been started; after 1,000 ml have been infused, the B/P is still low. The hospital team focuses on his low blood pressure and orders antishock trousers to be applied.

You decide to

1. refuse the order because of the chest injury
2. suggest trying dopamine first
3. apply the antishock trousers as ordered
4. immediately transport, "red light and siren"

Chest injury in a hypovolemic patient presents a relative contraindication when considering antishock trousers. That is, it is likely to cause an increase in intrathoracic pressure, which is undesirable in chest injuries. However, if the blood pressure cannot be controlled with rapid infusion of fluids, the antishock trousers may be required. The antishock trousers can be titrated to effect and the abdominal compartment deflated at the first sign of compromised respiratory efforts.

The antishock trousers are inflated, and the blood pressure is stabilized at 90 systolic. In the emergency room a chest tube is inserted to relieve a hemothorax. A belly tap is positive for gross blood in the abdomen, and surgery is performed to repair a lacerated liver.

The careful management of the unexpected in part determined how well we can provide patient care. Treatment protocols are an essential part of effective patient care, but they are only guidelines. Our success depends upon our ability to think and plan creatively and alternatively. We must constantly reevaluate our strategy as variable factors come into play.

The paramedic's on-site judgments are invaluable to the hospital team. They cannot see the patient, nor can they see the problems that the field team may be encountering.

As a final thought, and how often we have heard it, Don't forget the basics. When caring for multiple trauma patients, the ABCs are not just elementary, they are essential.

CASE STUDY 3B: MRS. D. WALLACE

You and your partner have just turned in for the night, hoping for an uneventful one. Sleeping straight through for six to eight hours is not common in your station, however, and tonight unfortunately will be no exception. The alarm sounds and the overhead lights burst on simultaneously. As driver, you write down the address on a notepad at the nearby desk and then quickly dress.

Your response is a short one to a mobile home park near the station. It's a retirement area that you visit frequently but, despite all your previous runs, the dark, narrow streets still confuse you. Your partner swings the spotlight up to illuminate addresses, and you stop at the appropriate mobile home. A man in his 60s meets you at the sliding glass door, and you both step into the living room.

Inside, reclining on a sofa, is your patient. She also appears to be in her late 60s and is quite pale, even in the low light of a table lamp. She has been feeling extremely weak all day long, her husband tells you, and had a brief "fainting spell" just before you were called. She is alert and her skin temperature feels normal. Her only medical problem is an occasional bout of indigestion, for which she takes Mylanta.

Which of the following symptoms concerns you most in this patient

1. generalized weakness
2. syncopal episode
3. indigestion
4. pale, warm, and dry skin

Syncope, while not uncommon in older patients, can result from any number of significant physiologic abnormalities. Among these are arrhythmias, hypotension, transient ischemic attacks, vagotonic reactions, and electrolyte imbalances. Further investigation of this patient's syncopal episode is definitely indicated.

Vital signs on your patient show that her pulse is 92 and regular, blood pressure is 146/78, and respirations are 18. The cardiac monitor is hooked up and shows a sinus rhythm with a normal P-R interval. On the basis of the circumstances surrounding her loss of consciousness, your partner decides to obtain orthostatic pulses and blood pressure while you make an initial report to the hospital.

Upon sitting up with her feet on the floor, the patient complains of some dizziness. In addition, the pulse increases to 120, and the blood pressure drops to 124/70. You place her in a supine position and give oxygen by mask. The monitor shows a sinus tachycardia.

This response should suggest

1. arrhythmia
2. transient ischemic attack
3. viral syndrome
4. hypovolemia

The response observed in this patient is consistent with a probable fluid loss (hypovolemia). Since there are no history of trauma and no reported overt blood loss, this should suggest the possibility of dehydration or internal bleeding. Further information on recent health problems or missed signs and symptoms should be considered.

Upon questioning the patient, you find that she had had some nausea but no vomiting in the past 24 hours. Her bowel movements have been regular, the stool normal in color and consistency. She has not had diarrhea and, until this morning, was eating normally. There is no history of cardiac disease or aneurysm. The hospital requests that you start an IV with lactated Ringer's to run at 200 ml/hour.

Which of the following would be appropriate to test for relative hypovolemia

1. fluid challenge with 250 ml of IV solution
2. apply antishock trousers with partial inflation
3. elevate the patient's lower extremities
4. any of the above followed by new vital signs

Actually, any of these techniques followed with updated vital signs can be effectively used to determine the presence of relative fluid loss. While this patient has no medical history to suggest otherwise, these tests would have to be used with extreme caution in patients with known cardiac or pulmonary insufficiency, such as congestive heart failure. In such patients, excess circulating volume is not well tolerated.

The hospital orders a fluid challenge for your patient. You are requested to open up the IV to run in 250 ml of lactated Ringer's solution. Your partner infuses the fluid and then takes another set of vital signs, with the patient first lying down and then sitting up. This time the patient feels better when she sits up, and her vital signs show a blood pressure of 140/72 and a pulse of 90. As you prepare to move her onto the gurney, however, she suddenly becomes very nauseated and vomits 200 to 300 ml of dark brown emesis.

This bloody emesis probably resulted from bleeding in the

1. colon
2. esophagus
3. liver
4. duodenum

Dark brown "coffee-ground" emesis results from gastric acids reacting with whole blood in the stomach. Bleeding from the stomach itself, or duodenal blood that has refluxed through the pyloris back into the stomach, will have this characteristic coffee-ground appearance when regurgitated. Esophageal blood is red, since it does not interact with stomach contents. Bleeding from other portions of the gastrointestinal (GI) tract generally shows up in the stool.

Your patient is loaded into the ambulance, and your partner continues to monitor her vital signs closely en route to the hospital. The IV is set at 200 ml/hour, and almost 350 ml have been infused upon your arrival at the emergency department.

Once in the ED, your patient is transferred to a waiting bed. The privacy curtain is drawn, and she is helped into a hospital gown while you brief the physician on her current status. The doctor expresses approval of your assessment and treatment and then disappears behind the curtain to examine the patient. Upon emerging, the doctor requests an electrocardiogram, complete blood count, electrolytes, platelet count, and prothrombin time.

Discussion

The GI tract proper extends from the stomach to the rectum. The esophagus is often included as part of this organ system and is itself subject to bleeding from varices, tumors, lacerations, etc. GI hemorrhage should be suspected especially in older patients with unexplained hypotension. Often, frank bleeding may not be present, and more subtle signs may present as a chief complaint. History is extremely important in these patients and can contribute to a rapid diagnosis. The patient may offer a history of previous ulcers, undiagnosed abdominal pain, syncope, alcoholism, tarry-colored stools, or previous GI hemorrhage. Obviously, gross blood vomited from the stomach or passed from the rectum determines the diagnosis.

Treatment is primarily supportive. Oxygen is always appropriate and should be given at moderate to high flow rates in a shocky patient. An IV with an isotonic crystalloid solution such as normal saline (ns) or lactated Ringer's (LR) is recommended. An IV catheter of 18 gauge or larger should be selected, because significant fluid replacement may be necessary. Orthostatic vital signs (lying and sitting or standing vital signs) and a fluid challenge can be helpful diagnostic tools to determine the presence of covert hypovolemia. For bleeding in the stomach, nasogastic suction should be considered. In rare cases of severe hypotension, antishock trousers should also be applied.

Upon gastroscopy, your patient is found to have a bleeding ulcer along the proximal wall of the duodenum. She is hospitalized for several days for observation and medical management.

RELATED ASSESSMENT QUESTIONS

3.1 Following completion of a venipuncture, to obtain a blood sample you should do all of the following *except*

- **(a)** be sure that the tourniquet has been released
- **(b)** label the container
- **(c)** hold the arm below the level of the heart
- **(d)** apply pressure to the site for three to five minutes
- **(e)** make sure that all bleeding has stopped

3.2 A scalp vein (butterfly) needle would be least appropriate for

- **(a)** elderly patients
- **(b)** pediatric patients
- **(c)** hypovolemic patients
- **(d)** patients with small veins
- **(e)** patients with respiratory congestion

3.3 How would you modify the antishock trousers application procedure to accommodate a patient who has a knife protruding from the abdomen:

- **(a)** position the suit so that its upper edge is just below the knife
- **(b)** remove the knife and apply the suit normally
- **(c)** apply the suit over the knife
- **(d)** don't apply the suit at all (use other antishock measures)
- **(e)** apply the suit normally, but don't inflate the abdominal compartment

3.4 Which of the following would be most appropriate for the field management of low-resistance shock:

- **(a)** IV fluids, sodium bicarbonate, and Aramine
- **(b)** epinephrine, IV volume expanders, and antishock trousers
- **(c)** IV TKO, antishock trousers, and possibly vasopressors
- **(d)** oxygen, semi-upright position, and IV fluids if needed
- **(e)** rotating tourniquets, IV fluids, and vasopressors

3.5 You have just started an IV but find that it is not running well. Blood has backed up and is continuing to rise in the tubing in a pulsating fashion. You suspect that you have inadvertently cannulated an artery. You should

(a) replace the IV tubing with a filtered blood administration set
(b) tape the needle securely in place, clamp off the flow of solution, and start a second IV
(c) remove the needle and apply pressure to the site for five minutes
(d) continue to use the IV as is, but watch closely for infiltration
(e) continue to use the IV for administration of solutions but not for any drugs

3.6 In order to start an IV on a cardiac arrest patient, you might try all of the following *except*

(a) apply a tourniquet
(b) elevate the legs
(c) apply antishock trousers
(d) give epinephrine subcutaneously
(e) lower the extremity

3.7 Large-bore IV cannulas are most appropriate for patients with

(a) cerebrovascular accidents (CVAs)
(b) febrile convulsions
(c) hypovolemic shock
(d) pulmonary edema
(e) anaphylaxis

3.8 Which of the following techniques would *not* be an appropriate way to distend the external jugular vein for insertion of an IV:

(a) compressing the vein above the clavicle
(b) applying antishock trousers
(c) elevating the legs
(d) lowering the head
(e) applying a tourniquet

3.9 When starting an IV, the tourniquet should be applied so that it

(a) occludes venous return but allows arterial flow
(b) occludes arterial flow but allows venous return
(c) impairs nerve impulses, thus reducing pain
(d) allows both arterial and venous flow
(e) occludes both arterial and venous flow

3.10 Which of the following is *not* an indication that the IV has infiltrated:

(a) swelling at the site
(b) inability to aspirate blood
(c) hematoma
(d) drip rate continually increasing
(e) no flashback of blood in tubing

3.11 How much solution does the pediatric IV administration set deliver:
(a) 1 microdrop per ml
(b) 5 microdrops per ml
(c) 10 microdrops per ml
(d) 30 microdrops per ml
(e) 60 microdrops per ml

3.12 In which of the following situations would you be *least* likely to use a volume control chamber (Volutrol) with the IV:
(a) for a child with febrile convulsions
(b) when Aminophylline is being given
(c) for a patient with congestive heart failure (CHF)
(d) when antishock trousers are needed
(e) when Physostigmine is being given

3.13 The most common complication associated with insertion of subclavian IV is pneumothorax. Which of the following would be *least* helpful in preventing this complication:
(a) place the patient in the shock position
(b) keep the patient well ventilated throughout the procedure
(c) tamponade the vein following removal of the needle
(d) keep all IV line connections secure
(e) ensure that all air is removed from the IV line

3.14 Which of the following is *least* likely to be included in the management of hypovolemic shock:
(a) oxygen
(b) IV fluids
(c) oral fluids
(d) shock position
(e) antishock trousers

3.15 Which of the following statements about the antishock trousers is true:
(a) they can't be used on pregnant women
(b) they are contraindicated in cardiac arrest
(c) they are applied so that the feet remain exposed
(d) they should be removed as soon as the BP returns to normal
(e) they cannot be used if CPR must also be performed

3.16 In which of the following is the antishock suit *least* likely to be indicated:
(a) cardiac arrest
(b) aneurysm
(c) gunshot wound to the abdomen
(d) pulmonary edema
(e) neurogenic shock

3.17 Prior to applying antishock trousers to a patient in shock, you should routinely
(a) assess lung sounds
(b) determine body weight

(c) insert an EOA
(d) suction the trachea thoroughly
(e) apply the cardiac monitor

3.18 Which of the following is an absolute contraindication to the use of anti-shock trousers:
(a) isolated head injury
(b) cardiogenic shock
(c) chest trauma
(d) pulmonary edema
(e) uncontrolled bleeding above the nipple line

3.19 Which of the following techniques will *not* help distend a vein for venipuncture:
(a) stroking the vein upward
(b) flicking lightly with two fingers
(c) elevating the extremity
(d) application of heat
(e) application of a tourniquet

3.20 How much solution does a standard IV administration set deliver:
(a) 10 drops per ml
(b) 15 drops per ml
(c) 20 drops per ml
(d) 25 drops per ml
(e) variable, depending on the manufacturer

3.21 You have 1 gm Lidocaine in 500 ml 5 percent D/W. What drip rate will you select to deliver 1 mg per minute if your infusion set delivers 60 microdrops per cc:
(a) 10 mcgtt/min
(b) 25 mcgtt/min
(c) 30 mcgtt/min
(d) 45 mcgtt/min
(e) 60 mcgtt/min

3.22 Which of the following signs/symptoms are *not* usually associated with shock:
(a) hypotension
(b) tachycardia
(c) decreased level of consciousness (LOC)
(d) cool, clammy skin
(e) depressed respirations

3.23 You have 1 gm Lidocaine in 250 ml 5 percent D/W with an IV set that delivers 60 microdrops per milliliter. You are ordered to set the rate to deliver 4 mg per minute. What drip rate will you select:
(a) 15 mcgtt/min
(b) 30 mcgtt/min
(c) 45 mcgtt/min

(d) 60 mcgtt/min
(e) 75 mcgtt/min

3.24 Syncope is very similar to other shock conditions, the primary difference being that syncope is
(a) much more severe
(b) only found in hysterical patients
(c) rare in children
(d) purely emotional and not a medical condition
(e) transient

3.25 Severe damage to the central nervous system causes a shock condition secondary to
(a) peripheral vasoconstriction with resultant cool, clammy skin
(b) peripheral vasodilatation with resultant "pooling" of blood
(c) loss of innervation to the heart with resultant cardiac failure
(d) tremendous blood loss from the brain substance into the cranium
(e) direct neuro-effect on the myocardium, causing increased heart rate

3.26 Neurogenic shock is best treated in the field with
(a) oxygen, IV, antishock measures, and prompt transport
(b) dopamine, IV fluids, and trendelenberg position
(c) IV fluids, Aramine, phlebotomy, and prompt transport
(d) oxygen, aggressive ventilation, and dopamine
(e) IV TKO, Levophed, antishock trousers, and oxygen

3.27 Hypovolemic shock should be treated with
(a) oxygen, analgesics, and slow IV fluids
(b) oxygen, rapid IV fluids, and antishock trousers
(c) analgesics, vasopressors, and transport
(d) oxygen and transport
(e) slow IV fluids, positioning, and transport

3.28 Cardiogenic shock should be treated in the field with
(a) EKG, slow IV, oxygen, and dopamine
(b) vasopressors, reassurance, rapid IV fluids, and transport
(c) analgesics, rapid IV fluids, oxygen, and EKG
(d) immediate transport without field treatment
(e) EKG, oxygen, elevated legs, and oral fluids

3.29 Anaphylactic shock should be treated in the field with
(a) antihistamines and rapid IV fluids
(b) IV, oxygen, and transport
(c) cricothyrotomy
(d) rebreathing bag, positioning, and epinephrine
(e) airway support, epinephrine, and antihistamines

3.30 Which of the following does *not* characteristically result in shock:
(a) heart's inefficiency as a pump
(b) blood loss

(c) peripheral "pooling" of blood
(d) blood pressure below 100 systolic
(e) inadequate perfusion

3.31 The blood pressure of a shock patient will
(a) always be low
(b) always be normal
(c) always be high
(d) frequently be low but may be normal
(e) frequently be normal but may be high

3.32 Perfusion is best described as
(a) distribution of oxygenated blood to the tissues
(b) rapid breathing
(c) good oxygenation of blood
(d) delivery of blood to the body tissues
(e) interruption of circulation

3.33 As the lumen of a blood vessel constricts and becomes narrower, the peripheral resistance will
(a) remain unchanged
(b) increase
(c) decrease
(d) increase only if blood volume is low
(e) decrease unless blood volume is low

3.34 The release of catecholamines (epinephrine and norepinephrine) helps to increase blood pressure by causing
(a) peripheral vasodilatation
(b) peripheral vasoconstriction
(c) increase in blood volume
(d) decrease in blood volume
(e) slowing of respirations

ANSWER KEY

3.1 c	**3.10** d	**3.19** c	**3.27** b
3.2 c	**3.11** e	**3.20** e	**3.28** a
3.3 e	**3.12** d	**3.21** c	**3.29** e
3.4 c	**3.13** b	**3.22** e	**3.30** d
3.5 c	**3.14** c	**3.23** d	**3.31** d
3.6 d	**3.15** c	**3.24** e	**3.32** a
3.7 c	**3.16** d	**3.25** b	**3.33** b
3.8 e	**3.17** a	**3.26** a	**3.34** b
3.9 a	**3.18** d		

4

GENERAL PHARMACOLOGY

CASE STUDY 4A: IV TRAINING DAY

You have been requested by the paramedic training center to help with training students on their "IV and Injection Technique" day. You, of couse, are merely present to instruct and not to offer yourself as a "patient" for these fledgling students. You can still recall your own anxiety about this phase of paramedic training and would swear that your novice partner that day used a 14-gauge IV cannula for his first "stick" on you.

You arrive promptly at the training class on the appointed morning. You find an empty seat near the rear of the room. First is a review of math used to calculate IV drip rates. You are inclined to doze because your help is obviously not yet needed, but for even an experienced paramedic the session dusts out a few mental cobwebs.

The first problem is an easy one. You are to find the drip rate to infuse 200 ml per hour of IV solution, using an IV set that delivers 15 drops (gtt) per ml. While the class works diligently with pencil and paper, you figure the problem quickly in your head.

The correct answer would be

1. 15 gtt/min
2. 25 gtt/min
3. 50 gtt/min
4. 200 gtt/min

Soon the instructor explains how to arrive at the proper answer of 50 gtt/min (see Table 4–1).

After several calculations for plain intravenous drips, the instructor moves to infusions of medications in dilution. First, the instructor covers proper labeling techniques for these solutions. Since these drugs are nearly always "piggybacked" into another IV line, labeling is of critical importance.

Which of these is *not* necessary information on such a label:

1. name of the medication
2. amount of drug added
3. paramedic's name or initials
4. rate of infusion

Because the rate at which a medication is being infused may vary, depending on the desired effect, this is usually not written on the label. In addition to the name and amount of drug added to the solution and the identification of the person who mixed it, the date and time of administration are also desirable.

Next there is some instruction on IV technique. Appropriate aseptic methods are discussed, then how to introduce an IV catheter into a vein.

"Now for the good part," you tell yourself. "Every paramedic should know just how much one of these needles can hurt."

The class splits into small groups, each student with a tourniquet and a handful of alcohol swabs. As you watch them practice, you try to emphasize things such as selecting a proper vein, placing the tourniquet, and stabilizing the vein before penetrating the skin. One student has introduced a cannula into a large vein of a classmate. The stylet is removed and the IV tubing is attached to the catheter hub, but there is no flow.

Which of the following would help the student determine whether the catheter is in the vein:

1. lower the solution container below the level of the IV site
2. reinsert the stylet and attempt to reposition the catheter
3. squeeze the IV bag and check for flow
4. place a tourniquet distal to the IV site

TABLE 4–1

Taking:	15 gtt./ml. × 200 ml./hr. = 3000 gtt./hr.
Then:	3,000 gtt./hr × 1 hr./60 min. = 50 gtt./min.

There are several reasons why an IV may not flow well. Lowering the IV bag or bottle below the level of the IV site and checking for blood return into the tubing is a simple and accurate method to determine proper placement of the cannula. Making sure that the tourniquet has been removed and looking for signs of infiltration near the site as well as kinks in the tubing are also important checks when an IV is running poorly or not at all.

After a lunch break, the class reconvenes for the afternoon session on injection techniques. Uses of various needle gauges and lengths are discussed along with intramuscular and subcutaneous methods of administration. As the students practice first on oranges and then on each other, you circulate from group to group, answering questions and giving tips on improving technique. The biggest difficulty for the students seems to be stabilizing the syringe and needle while aspirating to be certain that the medication (in this case sterile water) is not being given directly into a vein.

The major difference between intramuscular (IM) and subcutaneous (SQ) routes is that SQ injections are made

1. with 1/2- to 5/8-inch needle penetrating the skin at 90 degrees
2. with a 1- to 1 1/2-inch needle penetrating the skin at 45 degrees
3. with a 1- to 1 1/2-inch needle penetrating the skin at 90 degrees
4. with a 1/2- to 5/8-inch needle penetrating the skin at 45 degrees

The subcutaneous route is used by paramedics primarily in the administration of epinephrine (1:1,000) for the relief of bronchospasm. After the skin is prepped with an antiseptic swab, a short length (1/2 to 5/8 inch) needle is introduced at a 45 degree angle. Absorption of medications via this route is relatively rapid and predictable.

By now more than one student is complaining of the temporary effects of contusions and hematomas associated with IV and injection practice. The final topic of discussion will be intracardiac injections, and a model torso is brought out for demonstration purposes. There is a brief review of basic thoracic anatomy and how to locate and number the intercostal spaces. This route calls for a long intracardiac needle to be thrust through an intercostal space or just beneath the xyphoid into the ventricle, where inotropic drugs can be introduced directly into the heart.

Which of the following is the *least* likely complication with this technique

1. tissue embolus
2. cardiac tamponade
3. ventricular rupture
4. lacerated coronary artery

With intracardiac (IC) injections there is high risk of direct trauma to the heart itself, including cardiac tamponade, ventricular rupture, and laceration of a coronary artery. While introduction of a tissue embolus from the insertion of a large bore needle is possible, it is not a significant complication with this technique.

One by one the students practice an IC injection on the model, using several approaches with varying degrees of success. The class winds down and the students depart for the day, with a full evening of concentrated study ahead. You can remember how it was when you were a student and are sympathetic. For these motivated individuals, however, the personal discipline required to become a highly skilled and competent paramedic is not too high a price to pay.

CASE STUDY 4B: MR. P. FRANKLIN

Your paramedic unit is dispatched to an unconscious victim at a rock concert in an outdoor amphitheater. After parking as closely to the main gate as possible, you are approached by a security guard who tells you that there's a teenage male who passed out a few minutes ago. It could be drugs, but his friends say no. One of his men will take you to him.

As you and your partner follow closely behind the guard, you are bombarded with the sights, sounds, and odors unique to this kind of entertainment. Finally you reach the patient who is sprawled on the grass in front of the stage. He is totally unresponsive, and his breathing is very slow and shallow. His pulse is 56 and weak.

Initial treatment of this patient would probably not include

1. oropharyngeal airway
2. positive pressure ventilation
3. ammonia ampule
4. intravenous line

The initial care of any unconscious patient includes ensuring an adequate airway, effective ventilation, and circulation. Stimulating a patient with ammonia is appropriate in cases such as syncope and feigned unconsciousness. In these instances the patient should already have respirations and circulation that do not require additional support. This is obviously not true of your patient.

After inserting an oral airway, your partner begins ventilating the patient as you complete an initial assessment. The victim's blood pressure is 90/60 (taken by palpation): The skin is pale, warm, and dry; pupils are constricted and equal. There is no sign of head injury, and breath sounds are clear bilaterally. The cardiac monitor is also hooked up and shows sinus bradycardia. Since your EMS program permits initial envasive treatment to be started prior to contact with the hospital, you draw up 0.8 mg of Naloxone (Narcan) in a syringe to administer IM. With the Narcan quickly onboard you set up an IV with lactated Ringer's as your partner continues to manage the victim's airway.

Narcan, a narcotic antagonist, produces its pharmacologic effect by

1. inactivating any available narcotic in the bloodstream
2. competing with the narcotic for active receptor sites
3. stimulating the vital centers in the brain stem
4. the precise pharmacologic effect is unknown

Narcan is a pure narcotic antagonist, and it has virtually no adverse side effects. It has no effect in the absence of a narcotic since it reverses respiratory depression, hypotension, and coma associated with narcotic overdose by competitively binding to specific receptor sites. The onset of action is within two minutes, and its duration is 30 to 90 minutes.

With a patent IV line now established, you give an additional 0.4 mg of Narcan intravenously. Within moments the patient begins to regain consciousness and is now awake but confused. His blood pressure is 120/0, and the pulse rate is 104. He no longer requires positive pressure ventilation, and he pulls out the oral airway. With some assistance you and your partner manage to move your patient to the ambulance. Once inside the unit you note that his eyes are watering. He has a runny nose and is yawning frequently. He tells you that he is going to be sick to his stomach and that his skin itches.

These symptoms most likely indicate

1. narcotic withdrawal
2. an allergic response
3. amphetamine poisoning
4. two of the above

It is not unusual for administration of Narcan to a chronic narcotic user to result in withdrawal symptoms such as described here. Withdrawal occurs when the body has developed a physical dependence on the drug and then is deprived of a scheduled dosage. In addition, the patient may also become irritable and restless or may have a loss of appetite, nausea or vomiting, chills, or excessive sweating. A number of cardiac arrhythmias may also be observed.

Your patient continues to become increasingly restless and is fearful of getting busted for drug abuse. You speak calmly and reassure him of your willingness to help. His level of consciousness gradually deteriorates, and he becomes more difficult to arouse. Respirations have also become shallow. En route you administer another 0.4 mg Narcan IV and contact the hospital.

For which of these drugs would Narcan be least effective:

1. Darvon
2. heroin
3. dilaudid
4. cocaine

Although classified as a controlled substance, cocaine is neither an opium derivative nor synthetic and would not respond to this treatment.

Once at the emergency department your patient is closely observed, and a toxicology screen is performed to determine blood levels of narcotics and/or any other substances which might be present.

Discussion

Narcotic overdose is one of only a few acute drug poisonings that can be rapidly treated in the field. Narcotics are controlled substances and subject to scrupulous regulation owing to their high potential for dependance or addiction.

Narcotics are generally administered by injection or by mouth in tablet form and produce analgesia depressing the central nervous system. This effect reduces the patient's perception of pain. Additionally, these drugs can decrease motility of the GI tract, relieve anxiety, depress respiratory effort, and reduce blood pressure by vascular dilation.

In an overdose, narcotics characteristically produce decreased levels of consciousness, hypoventilation, and low blood pressure. Evidence of chronic use by injection may be present as track marks on the forearms, although other sites are commonly used.

Treatment includes airway management and assisting ventilations if necessary. An esophageal airway is not recommended for an apneic adult because rapid return of consciousness may result in its forceful removal by the patient. An intravenous line should be started with lactated Ringer's and Narcan given IM or, preferably, IV. The patient should also be on a cardiac monitor and be observed closely for recurrance of initial symptoms. All such patients should be seen in the Emergency Department.

Frequently, drugs may be mixed in an overdose, and, while narcotic effects may be reversed, other symptoms may persist. Narcan may be administered safely to any unconscious patient as a diagnostic step to rule out narcotic depression. If initial administration proves unsuccessful, a repeat dosage may be indicated followed in most case with 50 percent Dextrose.

Your teenage patient is a legally emancipated minor and refuses to be admitted to the hospital. Against medical advice, he signs a release of liability form and leaves the emergency department without follow up.

RELATED ASSESSMENT QUESTIONS

4.1 Which of the following steps is not appropriate when giving an IV push medication:
(a) ensuring that the IV line is patent
(b) applying a tourniquet
(c) obstructing IV flow above the injection site
(d) flushing tubing
(e) cleansing the site with an antiseptic pad

4.2 The most appropriate needle size for giving an IM injection is
(a) 18 gauge, 3/4 inch
(b) 23 gauge, 1 1/2 inch
(c) 21 gauge, 1 inch
(d) 25 gauge, 5/8 inch
(e) 16 gauge, 1/2 inch

4.3 An appropriate needle size for a subcutaneous injection is
(a) 18 gauge, 3/4 inch
(b) 23 gauge, 1 to 1/2 inch
(c) 21 gauge, 1 inch
(d) 25 gauge, 5/8 inch
(e) 16 gauge, 1/2 inch

4.4 Medications should not be given by the IM route to patients who
(a) are afraid of needles
(b) are in shock
(c) have had a CVA
(d) have a history of thrombophlebitis
(e) have readily accessible veins

4.5 Aminophylline is administered via IV Volutrol over a period of 20 to 30 minutes. To administer this drug in this manner, you would fill the Volutrol with about 50–100 ml of solution and then add how much Aminophylline:
(a) 100–200 mg
(b) 50–100 mg
(c) 1 gm
(d) 0.08 mg
(e) 250–500 mg

4.6 The *most* important question that you should ask prior to administering any kind of medication is
(a) "Are you a diabetic?"

(b) "Do you have any allergies?"
(c) "Do you have any medical insurance?"
(d) "Are you having any pain?"
(e) "Have you seen a private physician recently?"

4.7 While you are injecting medication directly into a vein, it is critical that you
(a) ask the patient if he or she has any allergies
(b) check frequently to see that you are still in the vessel
(c) watch the EKG for ectopics
(d) elevate the arm to enhance absorption
(e) check the blood pressure for adverse effects

4.8 You are ordered to add 1 gm of Lidocaine to an IV of 500 cc of D_5W and run it to administer 180 mg per hr. How fast would you have to run the IV:
(a) 4 microdrops per minute
(b) 30 microdrops per minute
(c) 60 microdrops per minute
(d) 65 microdrops per minute
(e) 90 microdrops per minute

4.9 You are ordered to give 3 mg of morphine intravenously. You have MS, 15 mg in 10 cc. How much will you give?
(a) 2 cc
(b) 1.4 cc
(c) 0.04 cc
(d) 0.2 cc
(e) 0.75 cc

4.10 Prior to giving any kind of an injection, you must do all of the following except
(a) apply a tourniquet
(b) cleanse the skin with antiseptic
(c) locate landmarks
(d) check for allergies
(e) aspirate for blood return

4.11 Which of the following routes of administration is fastest and most predictable:
(a) IM
(b) IV
(c) SQ
(d) sublingual
(e) oral

4.12 A systemic pharmacologic effect is one that acts on
(a) a specific body system
(b) one organ in a systematic way

(c) the body as a whole
(d) no more than one organ at a time
(e) all the organs in one system

4.13 Epinephrine and Isuprel have similar effects, so that when they both are given to the same patient, the effect is doubled. This is called
(a) multiplicity
(b) doubling effect
(c) cumulative effect
(d) synergistic effect
(e) antagonism

4.14 You are ordered tc give Valium 2.5 mg IV. You have 10 mg in 2 cc. You should inject
(a) 0.5 ml
(b) 1.0 ml
(c) 1.5 ml
(d) 2.0 ml
(e) 2.5 ml

4.15 You have 1 ml of epinephrine 1:1,000 in a syringe, but you need epinephrine 1:10,000. You can produce this concentration by
(a) discarding 0.5 ml
(b) adding 4 ml of saline
(c) adding 4 ml of saline and then discarding half the solution
(d) adding 9 ml of saline
(e) adding 9 ml of saline and then discarding half of the solution

4.16 Your patient weighs 150 pounds, and you need to give $NaHCO_3$ 1 mEq/kg. How much will you give:
(a) 68 mEq
(b) 75 mEq
(c) 93 mEq
(d) 128 mEq
(e) 132 mEq

4.17 You need nitroglycerine 15 mg. The bottle indicates that each tablet contains 1/4 grain. You should give
(a) 1/2 tablet
(b) 1 tablet
(c) 1 1/2 tablets
(d) 2 tablets
(e) 3 tablets

4.18 One tablespoon is equal to
(a) 3 cc
(b) 7.5 cc
(c) 10 cc

(d) 15 cc
(e) 30 cc

4.19 You need to give a 75 mg bolus of Lidocaine. You're out of the preloaded syringes, but you have 1 gm in a 50 ml vial in with your IV drugs. How much should you give:
- **(a)** 0.08 ml
- **(b)** 3.75 ml
- **(c)** 15 ml
- **(d)** 20 ml
- **(e)** none of the above; you can't use IV drip solutions as IV push drugs

4.20 IM injections usually begin to take effect in
- **(a)** 1 to 2 minutes
- **(b)** 5 to 10 minutes
- **(c)** 10 to 20 minutes
- **(d)** 30 minutes to 1 hour
- **(e)** 4 to 8 hours

4.21 When administering Isoproterenol by inhaler, it is important that you instruct the patient to
- **(a)** take a deep breath before spraying the drug
- **(b)** hold his or her breath once the drug has been inhaled
- **(c)** hyperventilate briefly after inhaling
- **(d)** hold the spray in his or her mouth before swallowing
- **(e)** breathe oxygen before and after inhaling the drug

4.22 In which of the following are you *least* likely to encounter adverse effects if Aminophylline is used:
- **(a)** children under 12 years of age
- **(b)** hypotensive patients
- **(c)** patients who take Theophylline preparations at home
- **(d)** hypoxic patients
- **(e)** patients who have pulmonary edema with associated wheezing

ANSWER KEY

4.1 b	**4.7** b	**4.13** c	**4.19** b
4.2 c	**4.8** e	**4.14** a	**4.20** b
4.3 d	**4.9** a	**4.15** d	**4.21** b
4.4 b	**4.10** a	**4.16** a	**4.22** e
4.5 e	**4.11** b	**4.17** b	
4.6 b	**4.12** c	**4.18** d	

5

RESPIRATORY EMERGENCIES

CASE STUDY 5A: CATHY A.

The tranquility of the pre-dawn darkness is broken by a two-tone station alarm, which drives slumbering firefighters from their bunks. ''Structure fire, 3256 Surrey Hill Place . . . time out: 0413 hours.''

From six blocks away, the dark sky is illuminated by a bright orange glow, which causes your heart rate to quicken. Once at the scene you methodically don a breathing apparatus while awaiting instructions from the engine company officer. As you momentarily study the two-story house, you can see flames spreading through a large broken window on the first floor. Upstairs is dark with only wisps of black smoke curling under the eaves.

''There may be a child inside,'' the captain's voice is edged with urgency. ''She was asleep in an upstairs bedroom. The rest of the family is out. You and Blackwood ladder the second-story window on the east side and make a search.''

The top of the ladder rests against the windowsill, and you climb the rungs to the closed window. To your surprise it slides open easily, and you carefully step into the darkness. Waiting for your partner to follow, you find your flashlight beam penetrates only a few feet into the smoke. Your partner, his voice muffled by his air mask, is soon crouched beside you. On hands and knees, you both begin to search the room. Near the floor the smoke is less dense, which allows somewhat better visibility. As you open a closet door, your flashlight illuminates a small, still form. Calling for your partner, you turn the child over. She is unconscious and her breathing is very slow and irregular.

Which of the following is the best course of action:

1. remove your air mask and perform mouth-to-mouth resuscitation
2. remove your air mask and place it over the child's face
3. move the patient outside immediately
4. have your partner inform the captain of the rescue

Removing your own mask while still exposed to a toxic atmosphere is never recommended. Although this patient obviously requires resuscitation, it cannot be effectively administered under such circumstances. The priority must be to move the patient to fresh air and proximity to resuscitation equipment. After completing this, you should inform the officer in charge as soon as possible.

Carefully lifting the child across your shoulder, you proceed to the window and down the ladder. Once on the ground, you gently lower the young girl to the grass. Quickly discarding your helmet, gloves, and air mask, you begin mouth-to-mouth breathing while awaiting oxygen equipment. A check of her carotid pulse gives you a rate of 140. She remains unconscious and unresponsive.

The probable physiologic cause of this patient's unconsciousness is

1. tissue irritation from smoke inhalation
2. respiratory burns from superheated air
3. metabolic acidosis following respiratory depression
4. hypoxia from carbon monoxide inhalation

Carbon monoxide's affinity for hemoglobin is 250 times greater than that of oxygen. When the oxygen-carrying capacity of blood is severely decreased by his combination of carboxyhemoglobin, the result is cerebral hypoxia, which produces a comatose state.

Your partner sets up the resuscitator and prepares to intubate the child with an endotracheal tube. She appears to be about six years old and approximately 45 pounds. After contact is made with the hospital, the ET tube is inserted on the first attempt, and good bilateral breath sounds are auscultated. Her blood pressure is 108/64, and small ventilations with a bag-mask are administered at a rate of 24 per minute. The EKG monitor shows a sinus tachycardia.

Which of these airway adjuncts would not be suitable for this patient

1. endotracheal tube
2. esophageal obturator airway
3. oral airway
4. pediatric bag mask with oxygen

The esophageal obturator airway is indicated only for airway management in an unconscious adult. While experimentation has been done on a pediatric version of the EOA, to date pediatric sizes are not available. It must be remembered that hypoxia is the primary cause of vomiting in an unconscious patient; thus, protecting the airway is of the utmost importance.

Respiratory burns must also be suspected and should be considered during patient assessment. Upon further examination, your patient appears to have no other injuries. The child's parents are standing nearby, anxious to know how their daughter is. You inform them that she will be taken to the hospital emergency room for further evaluation. The hospital requests that you continue ventilation, transport immediately and start an IV enroute.

Discussion

Victims of smoke inhalation are victims of carbon monoxide poisoning. Statistics reveal that some 80 percent of fire fatalities result from carbon monoxide poisoning. Since the normal combination of oxygen molecules with a hemoglobin molecule (oxyhemoglobin) is disrupted, the victim becomes hypoxic. Blood levels of carboxyhemoglobin (HbCO) can be measured and generally correlated with symptoms. Carboxyhemoglobin levels below 15 percent are generally asymptomatic. From 15 to 25 percent, the patient may complain of nausea, vomiting, dizziness, muscle weakness, and mental confusion. At 25 percent, hypoxic-related arrhythmias may appear, as well as extreme weakness and visual disturbances or blindness. HbCO concentrations of 40 percent or above produce unconsciousness; above 60 percent they are generally lethal.

Treatment is aimed at reducing carbon monoxide concentrations in the blood. Like radioactive materials, CO has a half-life, resulting from its tendency to combine with oxygen to form CO_2. Thus, oxygen therapy at high concentrations is indicated. Treating a patient with 100 percent oxygen reduces the half-life of carbon monoxide from 5 hours, 20 minutes to 1 hour, 20 minutes.

Optimal treatment of CO poisoning is carried out in a hyperbaric decompression chamber, where a patient can be given 100 percent oxygen at increased atmospheric pressure. This increases the partial pressure of oxygen in the blood and further enhances the elimination of carbon monoxide from the body.

In addition to CO poisoning, smoke inhalation can produce other complications. (Although generally not seen in the prehospital phase, they are presented here for completeness.) Exposure of lung tissue to toxic smoke and gases can produce pulmonary edema, pneumonia, and bronchitis.

Your patient regains consciousness in the emergency room, but remains hospitalized for several weeks following admission.

CASE STUDY 5B: MR. F. MITCHELL

Your paramedic unit is dispatched to a hotel in the downtown district for a man with breathing difficulty. When you pull up in front of the address you find a rather dilapidated old building in an area that traditionally attracts drunks and transients. You and your partner make your way up a dimly lit stairwell and down the hallway to a third-floor room. A knock on the door brings a faint response, and you both enter.

Inside is a man whom you estimate to be in his late 50s. He is sitting in a chair, leaning forward as he takes deep, rapid breaths. There are dozens of cigarette butts and numerous beer cans strewn about his ill-kept room. Your patient is dirty and his body odor is quite foul as your partner begins to examine him. He is conscious and alert, though apparently inebriated. His skin is pale, warm, and slightly moist. He tells you that he often has shortness of breath but that this episode began the night before and is worse than ever. He hasn't seen a doctor "in years" and takes no medications. Pulse is 120 and slightly irregular, respirations are 32 and labored, blood pressure is 162/90. Lung sounds reveal expiratory wheezing with fine rales in both bases. The EKG shows a sinus tachycardia with PACs, but the patient denies any chest pain. You note, however, that he is using some accessory muscles as he breathes, which accentuates his gaunt appearance.

Of the following choices, which do you consider most appropriate for this patient at this time:

1. oxygen, 2–4 l per cannula
2. oxygen, 8–10 l by mask
3. patient rebreathing into a paper bag
4. giving 100 percent oxygen by positive pressure ventilation

Most authorities agree that low flow oxygen (2–4 l per min) is at least initially adequate for a patient who is not clinically hypoxic (with cyanosis, mental confusion, etc.). This patient, though alert and without cyanosis, should benefit from oxygen by cannula.

After you secure the oxygen cannula in place, you go to the paramedic radio while your partner sets up the IV. The hospital responds to your initial assessment by ordering an IV of 5 percent D/W TKO. As you send an EKG strip, you summarily review several possible causes for this patient's condition.

Which would you *least* suspect to be the cause of his respiratory distress:

1. pneumonia
2. pleurisy
3. pulmonary edema
4. chronic obstructive pulmonary disease (COPD)

Pleurisy, an inflammation of the pleural lining, is generally characterized by sharp, inspiratory pain, which this patient denies. His medical history, though undiagnosed, suggests a chronic condition that results in dyspnea and shortness of breath. His age and poor overall physical condition make him a more likely candidate for unresolved pneumonia, pulmonary edema, or COPD.

The IV is established without difficulty, but the patient appears to have increasing difficulty in breathing. Your partner rechecks breath sounds and finds that there are increased wheezes on both sides with a prolonged expiratory phase.

Expiratory wheezes are most generally characteristic of:

1. bronchospasm
2. pulmonary edema
3. laryngitis
4. pneumonia

Wheezing, a sound generated by air being forced through constricted lower airways, is characteristic of bronchospasm and is frequently found in patients with COPD. Bronchospasm can also be present in acute congestive heart failure (CHF) patients resulting in "cardiac asthma."

You inform the hospital of your patient's increased dyspnea. You are concerned that this man may begin to deteriorate rapidly. He is slightly cyanotic and his respiratory rate is 40. The EKG and blood pressure are unchanged.

Which of the following drugs should you most expect the hospital to order:

1. atropine
2. epinephrine, 1:1,000
3. dopamine
4. aminophylline

It is very difficult to differentiate clinically between COPD and pulmonary edema in this patient. This is especially complicated by the fact that there is no definitive medical history available. Aminophylline, a potent bronchodilator, is most appropriate because it is useful for both bronchospasm caused by COPD and for pulmonary edema associated with congestive heart failure.

After a brief discussion with the hospital, you are ordered to administer Aminophylline, 250 mg in 50 ml of 5 percent D/W, IV Volutrol over 20 minutes. With Aminophylline infusing, you can ready this patient for transport to the hospital. En route your partner attempts to reevaluate the patient's lung sound to determine the effectiveness of the drug. Background noises in the ambulance make this especially difficult.

Suddenly your patient begins to become confused and uncooperative. His skin is very diaphoretic and cool. You glance at the monitor and see that his heart rate has fallen to 50 beats per minute. Respirations are 8 and labored. While your partner grabs the positive pressure valve and mask and begins to assist respirations, you immediately contact the hospital.

Which of the following is probably causing the patient's rapid decompensation:

1. irregular breathing pattern
2. oxygen overload
3. drop in cardiac output
4. hypoxia

While most of us have been trained to be cautious in the administration of oxygen to patients with COPD, the actual occurrence of apnea in these patients due to oxygen overload is relatively rare. Hypoxia due to pulmonary shunting and CO_2 retention more realistically leads to patient deterioration by producing a respiratory acidosis with concurrent changes in pO_2, pCO_2, and pH. Treatment of symptomatic arrhythmias and positive pressure ventilation are indicated.

The hospital requests continuous EKG telemetry and orders atropine, 0.5 mg IV. You take over ventilating the patient, while your partner gives the atropine IV push. Your patient is unconscious but responds to verbal stimulus by mumbling incoherently. As you arrive at the emergency room, the monitor shows his heart rate to be 72. The patient is transferred to the hospital gurney, and blood gases are drawn as the emergency room physician intubates his trachea. An additional 250 mg of Aminophylline is infused before significant relief is observed.

Discussion

Chronic lung disease should always be considered in dyspneic patients over 45 years old. Oxygen administered in low flow rates is recommended because higher concentrations paradoxically can cause increasing acidosis in patients who rely on a hypoxic drive. Since these patients can deteriorate very rapidly, a keep-open IV line, monitor, and prompt transport are always indicated. Respiratory depressants such as morphine and Valium are obviously contraindicated. For this reason, utmost caution must be exercised when differentiating between COPD and pulmonary edema.

Owing in part to prompt prehospital care, your patient is released from the hospital two weeks after admission for COPD.

CASE STUDY 5C: MRS. A. GARCIA

You respond to a request for paramedics at a local bank during regular business hours. As you arrive in front, the bank president meets you and tells you that one of his loan officers has severe chest pain. He is sure that she is having a heart attack.

Once inside the bank, you are led to the employees' lounge where you find a woman in her mid-40s sitting in a chair. She is, in fact, having severe chest pain, which developed suddenly while she was working on an account. She describes it as a sharp pain right beneath her sternum, which seems to worsen when she takes a deep breath. She appears very anxious and is markedly short of breath. There is no history of cardiac disease, but you note that she is overweight. She tells you that she had a hysterectomy four weeks ago and is taking Premarin. At this point, you decide that the most likely cause for this patient's chest pain is

1. acute myocardial infarction
2. pulmonary embolus
3. dissecting aneurysm
4. unknown, more information needed

The danger of jumping to a premature diagnosis is obvious. You may miss important history or perform an inadequate physical exam. While there is nothing wrong with maintaining a working diagnosis, we must avoid being trapped by tunnel vision. It is important to treat symptomatically and cautiously.

Your assessment further reveals that the patient has pale, cool, and moist skin. Her pulse is 136, respirations are 36 and shallow, and B/P is 136/100. Lung sounds are clear bilaterally. The monitor shows a sinus tachycardia with 6 to 8 (PVCs) a minute. As you finish your physical exam, your partner puts her on oxygen at 8 l by nasal cannula. Premature ventricular contractions are considered dangerous in the presence of chest pain because

1. they do not perfuse blood adequately
2. they indicate the presence of cardiac irritability
3. they can lead to lethal ventricular arrhythmias
4. all of the above

PVCs are indicative of cardiac irritability. They are considered dangerous because they do not perfuse well and because they often lead to ventricular tachycardia or fibrillation. Although PVCs are often a result of hypoxia and may be eliminated by administration of oxygen, ventricular ectopics that occur in the presence of chest pain should be watched closely and treated prophylactically with Lidocaine.

After contacting the hospital, you are ordered to start an IV with 5 percent D/W TKO. Your first attempt to start the IV is unsuccessful. A second try finds the elusive vein, and the IV flows well. The hospital orders Lidocaine to be administered, 1 mg per kg IV push, to be followed with a 50 mg bolus every 10 minutes to a maximum of 225 mg. Given the above therapeutic dosage of Lidocaine, what desirable effect can you expect to see within 1 to 2 minutes:

1. an increase in heart rate
2. a decrease in ventricular ectopics
3. an increase in blood pressure
4. a decrease in anxiety level

Normal onset of effect for Lidocaine can be expected within two minutes and should be observed as a decrease in ventricular ectopic beats. *Caution:* Allergies to local anesthetics such as Novocain, Carbocaine, and Xylocaine are common. Always obtain a history of possible allergies prior to administration. The schedule of repeated bolus administration should eliminate the need to start an IV Lidocaine drip prior to arrival at the hospital.

Your patient continues to be cool and increasingly diaphoretic. Her skin color is slightly cyanotic. A quick recheck of her vital signs shows a weak pulse of 148, respirations of 38 and labored, and blood pressure of only 90/60. She is also becoming confused and combative.

Acute onset of shock in this patient can realistically only be hypovolemic or cardiogenic in nature. Since volume replacement would be contraindicated in cardiogenic shock, it is important to determine the cause of the shock state if possible. Of the following procedures, which would most quickly determine the presence of pump failure:

1. auscultate heart sounds
2. sit the patient up and check for neck vein distention

3. check bilateral pulses and blood pressures
4. perform a fluid challenge

Distention of the neck veins in a patient who is sitting up is an excellent diagnostic tool in determining pump failure. Though commonly seen in CHF, neck vein distention is often present in cardiogenic shock. It further shows that fluid replacement is not indicated.

Upon exam you will find that your patient does, in fact, have markedly distended neck veins proceeding from the angel of the jaw to the midclavicular point. You determine that this patient is probably in cardiogenic shock. The most appropriate treatment for this shock condition would be

1. dopamine titrated to blood pressure
2. antishock trousers
3. high flow oxygen and elevated lower extremities
4. IV solution switched to Ringer's or normal saline

Dopamine is the drug of choice in cardiogenic shock and is indicated to maintain blood pressure in shock states after sufficient volume replacement, if necessary, has been achieved. Vasopressors such as Aramine or Levophed may also be appropriate under these conditions.

You receive an order to hang a dopamine drip en route and transport stat. The patient is placed on the gurney and wheeled quickly to the waiting ambulance. Once inside you realize how hard you have been working. As your partner labels and then piggybacks the second IV bag into the line, you get another blood pressure reading. It is 60/0 by palpatation. You try to maintain her B/P at 90 to 100 systolic.

Cardiogenic shock may be caused by

1. myocardial infarction
2. pericardial tamponade
3. pulmonary embolus
4. any of the above

Cardiogenic shock can be recognized by the onset of hypotension, which results from acute pump failure. Any of these conditions may cause it, because cardiac output is severely compromised by overload, tamponade, or large loss of myocardial tissue due to infarct. This condition carries a high risk of mortality, and, thus, immediate transport is mandatory.

Upon arrival at the hospital, the ER staff is waiting. The physician performs a rapid exam and orders arterial blood gases (ABGs), portable chest X-ray, and 12-lead EKG. ABGs reveal severe pulmonary insufficiency, indicative of a large pulmonary embolus. The patient is started on Heparin and high flow oxygen in the ER and is transferred to the intensive care unit.

Prompt transport by the paramedics and a rapid diagnosis by the emergency room physician contribute to this patient's slow but eventual recovery.

Chest pain, regardless of its cause or the patient's age, must always be considered significant. Though obviously not always cardiac in etiology, these patients warrant close monitoring of EKG and vital signs as well as prompt transport. A thorough physical exam should always be performed, rapidly but without shortcuts. Treatment should be aimed at airway management, relief of anxiety, control of cardiac arrhythmias, and analgesia, if indicated.

CASE STUDY 5D: MR. L. LAZZARO

"Rescue 1, respond to a vehicle accident with injuries, on the Evergreen Highway near mile marker 3. Alpine Ambulance en route, time out: 1632." As your fire department's quick-attack rescue rig clears the station, you are reminded of countless runs up this steep highway into the mountainous terrain west of town. There have been many serious auto accidents with an always critical 30- to 45-minute transport time to the hospital. For the moment there seems to be no immediate solution to this frequently encountered problem of your rural EMS system.

Arriving at the scene, you see an ominous set of fresh skid marks leading to a splintered guardrail overlooking a steep canyon. Some 200 feet down the steep embankment you see an automobile resting on its side. By radio you request an additional engine company from a neighboring township. In the distance you can hear the siren of the approaching ambulance. You order two ropes to be tied off and cast down the slope for a controlled descent to the wreckage. Before descending with your partner, you ask the remaining two firefighters to prepare the Stokes stretcher to be lowered to you with a resuscitator, drug box, cervical collars, and monitor. You and your partner adjust your mountaineering harness, clip into the two ropes, and start down the slope. Upon reaching the car, you hear a voice moaning inside.

As your first priority you would

1. check for a leaking fuel tank
2. shatter a window and enter the car
3. make certain that the vehicle is stable
4. initiate radio contact with the hospital

One of the first rules of automobile extrication is always to make certain that the vehicle is stabilized. This is especially important with an automobile on its side because the center of gravity is high and weight distribution is altered. Wooden cribbing and ropes must be utilized to secure the auto in its present position prior to entering the vehicle for patient assessment.

The sedan rests on its side with the roof facing uphill. Ropes are quickly tied off to the front and rear bumpers; short sections of 2-by-4 lumber are used to construct a "crib" under the downhill side of the vehicle. As you look inside the car from the rear, there appears to be a single occupant in the front seat. The rear window of tempered glass is quickly disintegrated with a spring-loaded centerpunch. As your partner climbs through the rear window to examine the patient, you ask to have an air chisel sent down in order to gain access through the vehicle's vulnerable roof. From inside the car your partner relays his initial assessment to you. The patient is a male in his late 20s. He is conscious and alert. He is short of breath and complains of right-sided chest pain, which is worse when he takes a deep breath. He also has an open fracture of his right lower leg. His pulse is 120 and regular, respirations are 28 and labored, blood pressure is 136/88.

What should be the next step in your assessment of this patient

1. skin color, moisture, and temperature
2. abdominal check
3. pulses distal to the leg fracture
4. breath sounds

A complete head-to-toe exam should always be performed so that important findings are not missed. While all the findings are significant in the assessment of this patient, the most important initial finding in any trauma patient who has chest pain with shortness of breath is an evaluation of breath sounds.

Your partner informs you that breath sounds are clear in the left lung field and possibly diminished in the lower right. The skin is moist and cool. Bleeding from the open fracture is minimal, and the patient's abdominal findings are negative. The resuscitator is passed through the rear window to your partner, who puts the patient on oxygen by mask. The air chisel extrication tool has been sent. The car's sheet metal roof is quickly opened on three sides and folded down. Inside, two support members are cut and the vinyl headliner is ripped open, exposing your partner and his patient. The patient has no neck or back pain; however, as a routine precaution, a cervical collar is put around his neck. After a sterile dressing is placed on the open wound, a ladder splint is used to immobilize the leg fracture. The operation goes smoothly as the patient is strapped securely into the Stokes basket and transferred up the hill to the waiting ambulance.

Which of these choices do you consider *inappropriate* for this patient

1. prompt transport
2. morphine, slow IV for chest pain
3. re-evaluation of respiratory status
4. IV with lactated Ringer's

As a rule, any patient with impaired respiratory status secondary to trauma should always be transported without delay. In this patient, an IV is indicated but may be started en route. Morphine is contraindicated because of impending shock and the drug's depressive action on respiratory function.

Once in the ambulance your partner reevaluates the patient. He is pale, cool, and moist and is becoming more dyspeneic. Lung sounds are still diminished in the right lower lung field. He is on oxygen at 8 l by mask. An IV is started in the patient's left arm with a large-bore cannula. You are en route to the nearest hospital with an estimated time of arrival (ETA) of 25 minutes. Other than the leg fracture, a rapid secondary exam reveals no other significant injuries. Vital signs are pulse 136, respirations 36 and labored, B/P 120/90. You suspect that your patient has a probable pneumothorax on the right side.

All of the following signs are suggestive of a developing tension pneumothorax except

1. distant heart sounds
2. marked increasing dyspnea
3. distended neck veins
4. hyper-resonance to percussion

A tension pneumothorax can result when the chest wall or the lung itself is perforated. The patient's dyspnea increases markedly as air enters the interpleural space on inspiration but cannot escape on expiration. Intrathoracic pressure continues to build, leading to severely compromised cardiac output and shock. Distant heart sounds, rarely discernible in the field, are indicative of cardiac tamponade.

Your patient begins to show signs of increased breathing difficulty. The chest wall is tender on palpation. There is no apparent paradoxical breathing to suggest a flail chest, and the EKG shows a sinus tachycardia. Breath sounds are definitely absent in the right chest. The patient is becoming cyanotic and combative. The hospital is still 15 minutes away, but radio communication is possible. After updating the ER physician on the patient's status, you request permission to perform a needle thoracostomy. After carefully prepping the site at the right second intercostal space in the midclavicular line, you insert the trochar and note a wisp of air escaping through the one-way valve.

Upon arrival at the emergency room, your patient has improved considerably. His respirations are still 28 and shallow, but skin color is normal. A portable X-ray reveals fractured ribs on the right side. Blood gases, type and crossmatch, as well as urinalysis are also done. A chest tube is inserted in the ER, and the patient is sent to surgery. After open reduction of the fractured tibia and fibula, the patient is sent to intensive care in serious condition.

Trauma to the chest often presents a grave prognosis because cardiac or respiratory functions are frequently affected. Field treatment is limited in most cases, and surgery may be indicated. Primary consideration must be given to airway, breathing, and circulation (as always) along with prompt assessment and transport. Oxygen should always be administered (by mask if tolerated). An IV with Ringer's lactate or normal saline should be started because of risk of hypovolemia; however, transport should not be delayed. Monitoring the patient's EKG is important because cardiac contusion, infarct, or tamponade can produce arrhythmias. Remember that any chest wound below the nipple line is also a potential abdominal injury.

Your patient responds well to treatment and is discharged from the hospital four weeks later.

CASE STUDY 5E: MS. M. THORNTON

One of those ideal "get-away-from-it-all" vacations is rare for you in your work as an EMT-Paramedic. Although your 24-hour shift schedule does permit time away from the job, continuing education, family commitments, and other responsibilities seem to have consumed most of your spare time. For months you have anticipated a week of rest and recreation in the Colorado Rockies. You and your spouse are both avid joggers, experienced in the outdoors, and intend to backpack to a remote mountain lake at the 10,500 foot level. It is early October, and, though you are prepared for cold weather, you anticipate clear days and warm temperatures.

Your ascent from the trail head is rigorous but not exhausting, and within a few hours you are gazing at a breath-taking panorama. As you begin to pitch camp, your spouse points out the presence of another hiking party whose orange tent is visible across the lake. After a light lunch you decide to hike around to meet your neighbors, who, to your mutual delight, turn out to be a very amiable couple in their mid-40s. They had arrived the previous evening and also intend to stay for several days.

Darkness comes early in the high country, and not long after you have retired to your tent you hear a voice just outside. "Are you asleep? We need your help." It is the voice of the man across the lake. "It's my wife, She's very sick."

Accompanying your friend back to his camp, you and your spouse listen intently. "An hour or so ago she started to feel very weak all over. She didn't want any dinner, and she crawled into her sleeping bag to rest. I figured she was just exhausted from yesterday's climb. Then she started to cough and gasp for breath. Since you are a paramedic, I thought you would know what to do."

As you and your spouse slip into the small tent, you are alarmed by the woman's appearance. Her skin is pale and feels warm and dry. Her respirations 32 and slightly labored. Her pulse rate is 135 and regular. She is alert and complains of generalized weakness, headache, and a dry cough. She describes a feeling of tightness in her chest but has no chest pain. She has no previous medical problems and takes no medications.

Given this history and physical findings you might suspect

1. cardiac dysrhythmia
2. acute allergic reaction
3. high altitude sickness
4. all of the above

Each of the above diagnoses can produce the symptoms given; however, high altitude sickness should be suspected whenever an unacclimatized person becomes acutely ill or listless above 8,000 feet.

Symptoms of high altitude sickness are unlikely to occur below 8,000 feet in elevation. Severe cases can result in high altitude pulmonary edema (HAPE) and/or high altitude cerebral edema (HACE), either of which may cause death if not treated. In any event, immediate descent for medical treatment is indicated.

It is expected that your patient's condition will continue to deteriorate if she remains at this altitude. Systematically you begin to weigh critical factors in your mind:

Terrain: good trail, steep descent.
Time of Day: 2000 hours (8 PM), darkness, no moon, first light not expected for 10 hours.
Weather: clear and cool.
Patient's condition: worsening.
Distance to Trail Head: six miles.
Nearest Available Medical Care: rural hospital 35 miles away.

Which of the following alternatives would you now select:

1. stay put and monitor the patient's condition until dawn
2. plan an immediate descent to lower altitude with the patient
3. attempt to hike out alone in order to summon aid
4. reassure the patient that her condition may improve within the next 12 hours

Obviously you are faced with a most difficult decision. Since it is unlikely that your patient's condition will improve and that delaying treatment will be injurious, hiking out with the patient is the best remaining option. Even a descent of a few thousand feet may produce significant improvement for the patient and should be initiated with utmost attention to safety.

As you and the husband prepare a makeshift litter by stretching a sleeping bag between two aluminum tent poles, your spouse watches the patient carefully. She is having increasingly labored respirations and has some peripheral cyanosis. Her pulse rate is 140, and her coughing now produces a white, frothy sputum. In addition, she speaks little and is becoming less cooperative. Your spouse encourages her to take full, deep breaths.

The patient's deteriorating condition is most likely a direct result of

1. pulmonary congestion
2. cardiogenic shock
3. congestive heart failure
4. hypertension

The most reasonable explanation for the patient's breathing difficulty, frothy sputum, and abnormal behavior is pulmonary congestion caused by fluid in the lungs; that is, pulmonary edema. This results in severe hypoxia because venous blood is poorly oxygenated in the pulmonary capillary beds.

After placing the woman on top of the litter, the four of you begin the descent. Going down with her feet first enables you to keep the patient's head elevated, thus slightly assisting her ventilation. Though your patient is not heavy, the increased exertion at a high altitude forces all of you to stop frequently to catch your breath. With each stop you check the patient. Audible congestive sounds heard with each breath she takes confirm your suspicion that she has developed high altitude pulmonary edema. It is frustrating to know that there is little you can do for her. Your spouse, who is a critical care nurse, rechecks respirations, which are 40, and the pulse rate, which is 138 and slightly irregular.

Although there is no cardiac monitor at hand, which of these arrhythmias would least likely produce the observed pulse:

1. mobitz 1 (Wenchbach)
2. atrial fibrillation
3. sinus tachycardia with PVCs
4. atrial flutter with 3:1 block

It should be remembered that although a presumptive diagnosis has been made, other possibilities do exist. Because the patient is clinically hypoxic, the rhythm you might likely expect would be a sinus tachycardia with premature beats. Only atrial flutter with a constant 3:1 block would not produce an irregular pulse.

It takes nearly eight hours to reach the trail head. Your patient has shown little improvement, though she is no worse. After loading her into your four-wheel drive vehicle, you proceed directly to the hospital nearly 35 miles away. Once in the small emergency room, arterial blood gases and a chest X-ray are performed. She is then given positive pressure breathing treatment and admitted to the hospital for several days of observation.

Discussion

High altitude sickness can manifest itself in a number of different ways. It can be easily confused with other illnesses and cannot be ruled out on the basis of patient's age, sex, or level of fitness. There is no reliable way to predict who might be affected. Symptoms are most generally related to increasing cerebral edema and/or pulmonary edema, which occur within 12 to 36 hours. Early signs of high altitude sickness include light-headedness, headache, nausea and vomiting, and anorexia (loss of appetite). As the illness continues to progress, symptoms such as generalized weakness, ataxia (loss of coordination), coughing, and shortness of breath during mild exertion may develop. In severe cases the victim may become apathetic, confused, or even unconscious. Coughing may also produce white or pink-tinged frothy sputum as decreased atmospheric pressure in the alveoli allow for diffusion of fluids from the capillaries.

Treatment is two-fold: First, high altitude sickness is most often associated with rapid ascent to above 8,000 feet without adequate acclimatization. Although oxygen concentration is 21 percent regardless of the elevation, air is less dense the higher the altitude. This means that a larger volume of gas must be inhaled to achieve the same relative oxygen saturation in the blood; consequently, people breathe rapidly and more deeply at higher altitudes. For this reason, prevention is focused on spending more time while ascending, which allows for physiological adaptation. Early symptoms must not be ignored. Second, in moderate to severe cases immediate descent is the treatment of choice. Oxygen should be used if available. In all but mild cases the patient should be encouraged to be seen by a physician.

While not seen commonly by most prehospital care teams, this illness must be expected whenever treating someone who has been at higher elevations (for example, hikers, campers, skiers, or fliers). A basic understanding of the physiology involved can also be most helpful.

Your patient is discharged home for recuperation after four days thanks to your aid. Meanwhile, you and your spouse return to the high country to enjoy your well-earned rest.

RELATED ASSESSMENT QUESTIONS

5.1 Your patient is a 23-year-old male suffering an acute onset of shortness of breath, accompanied by a sharp pain in his left shoulder, which is aggravated by breathing. Lung sounds are clear, although they seem somewhat diminished on the left side. These findings are suggestive of
(a) pulmonary edema
(b) spontaneous pneumothorax
(c) asthma
(d) anaphylactic shock
(e) acute myocardial infarction

5.2 Which of the following is *not* a contraindication to insertion of an esophageal airway:
(a) foreign body obstruction of the upper airway
(b) overdose known to be caused by heroin
(c) massive facial trauma
(d) abdominal distention
(e) pediatric patients

5.3 Carbon monoxide poisoning is best treated by
(a) hyperventilation with 100 percent oxygen
(b) breathing into a paper bag
(c) 50 mg carboxyhemoglobin IV push
(d) low flow oxygen
(e) 25 mg Benadryl IV push

5.4 The Magill forceps is used in conjunction with a laryngoscope to
(a) insert an endotracheal tube
(b) remove foreign body obstructions of the upper airway
(c) perform a cricothyrotomy on an unconscious patient
(d) insert an esophageal airway
(e) insert a nasogastric tube

5.5 Which of the following is *not* consistent with the typical clinical picture of tension pneumothorax:
(a) cyanosis
(b) increasing dyspnea
(c) absence of breath sounds
(d) muffled heart sounds
(e) tracheal deviation

5.6 When performing a needle thoracostomy to relieve a tension pneumothorax, you must be sure that the cannula is securely connected to the
(a) one-way flutter valve
(b) main-line IV
(c) EKG monitor

(d) suction apparatus
(e) oxygen tubing

5.7 In which of the following are rales *least* likely to be heard:
(a) laryngeal edema
(b) asthma
(c) pulmonary edema
(d) near-drowning
(e) IV fluid overload

5.8 When epinephrine is given SQ for an adult asthma patient, the proper dosage is
(a) 0.1 mg
(b) 0.3 mg
(c) 1 mg
(d) 8 mg
(e) 10 mg

5.9 Following a traffic accident, your patient complains of sharp pain on inspiration. The patient has absent breath sounds unilaterally. You suspect that the patient has
(a) foreign body obstruction
(b) pericardial tamponade
(c) pulmonary embolus
(d) asthma
(e) pneumothorax

5.10 Which of the following would *not* be an appropriate treatment for a patient suspected of having a hemothorax:
(a) control external bleeding
(b) give MS to relax respiratory effort
(c) start an IV of RL or NS
(d) give high flow oxygen; ventilate if needed
(e) stabilize chest wall as needed

5.11 Your patient is found in an apartment; symptoms include dry cough, pain on inspiration, headache, mental sluggishness, and generalized muscle tremors. Dyspnea seems to be getting worse. Which of the following would be first on your list of suspicions:
(a) CHF
(b) gas inhalation
(c) pulmonary embolus
(d) asthma
(e) acute MI

5.12 The most common and most easily prevented side effect of tracheal suctioning is
(a) reflex bradycardia
(b) aspiration

(c) hypoxia
(d) ventricular irritability
(e) damage to mucous membranes

5.13 Your patient has an esophageal obturator airway in place but has regained consciousness and is fighting the airway. You have tried to explain the situation to the patient, but the patient continues to gag on the airway. You should:
(a) sedate the patient
(b) replace the EOA with an ET tube
(c) give the patient Lidocaine to suppress the gag reflex
(d) apply soft restraints and leave the airway in place
(e) remove the EOA and suction if necessary

5.14 When tracheal suctioning is performed, the suction is applied
(a) only during insertion of the catheter
(b) only while the catheter is at the carina
(c) only while removing the catheter
(d) both during the insertion and during removal of the catheter
(e) at any point; it doesn't make any difference

5.15 The metabolic acidosis that accompanies *prolonged* respiratory arrest is best treated with artificial respiration and
(a) Aminophylline
(b) sodium bicarbonate
(c) calcium chloride
(d) Isuprel
(e) Lasix

5.16 In which of the following situations would an endotracheal tube be contraindicated:
(a) laryngeal edema
(b) foreign body obstruction of the upper airway
(c) respiratory depression
(d) pediatric patients
(e) cardiac arrest

5.17 Which of the following is an indication for the use of Aminophylline:
(a) ventricular irritability
(b) asthma
(c) organophosphate poisoning
(d) hypotension
(e) seizures

5.18 The field dosage of sodium bicarbonate is determined by body weight. Which of the following parameters should also be considered:
(a) arterial blood gases
(b) skin color
(c) blood pressure

(d) respiratory status
(e) level of consciousness

5.19 In attempting to remove a foreign body obstruction from an airway, you would *not* use the Magill forceps unless you
(a) started an IV and monitored the EKG
(b) got a signed consent form
(c) first checked the blood pressure
(d) could visualize the larynx
(e) also inserted an oropharyngeal airway

5.20 Which of the following should be avoided when treating an asthmatic:
(a) epinephrine
(b) Benadryl
(c) Isuprel
(d) Aminophylline
(e) high flow oxygen

5.21 Following insertion of the EOA, you should always
(a) auscultate chest bilaterally
(b) give high flow oxygen
(c) check for presence of gag reflex
(d) suction trachea via the EOA
(e) insert a nasogastric tube

5.22 A common complication of endotracheal intubation is aspiration of chipped tooth fragments. This can largely be prevented by
(a) keeping the laryngoscope blade off the teeth
(b) padding the teeth with a rolled towel
(c) suctioning the mouth continuously during the procedure
(d) placing a strip of adhesive tape across the top of the teeth
(e) all of the above

5.23 Whenever an esophageal airway is removed, you should be prepared immediately to
(a) ventilate the patient
(b) suction the patient
(c) notify the hospital
(d) give sodium bicarbonate
(e) replace it with an ET tube

5.24 You have determined that your patient is experiencing hyperventilation syndrome. Your most appropriate action is to
(a) have the patient breathe into a paper bag
(b) give 250 mg Aminophylline IV Volutrol
(c) give high flow oxygen by mask
(d) ventilate with positive pressure ventilator
(e) start an IV and transport

5.25 Which of the following would be *least* suggestive of a respiratory burn:
(a) soot around nose and mouth
(b) dyspnea
(c) singed nasal hairs
(d) blisters around the mouth
(e) Cheyne-Stokes respirations

5.26 Your patient is experiencing difficulty breathing and has copious, frothy sputum. The patient is cyanotic and has distended neck veins; B/P is 176/96, pulse 146, and respirations 44. This clinical picture is characteristic of
(a) pulmonary edema
(b) carbon monoxide poisoning
(c) drug-induced respiratory insufficiency
(d) hyperventilation syndrome
(e) smoke inhalation

5.27 Which of the following is the correct dosage for the *initial* dosage of sodium bicarbonate during a cardiac arrest:
(a) 50–100 mEq IV or IC
(b) 500 ml 25 percent IV drip
(c) 2–10 units IV push
(d) 1 mEq per kg IV push
(e) 15–20 mg per kg IV push

5.28 Which of the following would be *least* helpful in opening an airway that has been completely occluded by a foreign body:
(a) Heimlich maneuver
(b) 100 percent oxygen
(c) chest thrusts
(d) Magill forceps and laryngoscope
(e) repositioning the head

5.29 One of the most important precautions to be taken while using the EOA is
(a) selection of correct size
(b) suctioning during insertion
(c) auscultation after insertion
(d) avoiding use during CPR
(e) removal after 15 minutes

5.30 Your patient is a 16-year-old who has just been involved in a family argument. The presenting clinical picture includes dizziness, tachypnea, numbness around the mouth, and tingling in the fingertips. You suspect:
(a) Valium overdose
(b) asthma
(c) neurological palsy

(d) hyperventilation syndrome
(e) seizure disorder

5.31 Rotating tourniquets can be used to treat the patient who is in
(a) hemorrhagic shock
(b) diabetic ketoacidosis
(c) right-sided heart failure
(d) status asthmaticus
(e) pulmonary edema

5.32 Which of the following will *not* assist in opening the airway:
(a) hyperextend the neck and pull the jaw forward
(b) insert an oral airway
(c) suction the mouth and oropharynx
(d) insert a nasogastric tube
(e) insert an endotracheal airway

5.33 You encounter a patient with foreign body obstruction of the upper airway. The patient has inspiratory stridor and is in severe respiratory distress. The patient is still coughing forcefully; therefore, you should:
(a) leave the patient alone and see if the patient can dislodge it
(b) perform 6 to 10 manual thrusts
(c) use a Choke-Saver to remove the obstruction
(d) use a Magill forcep and laryngoscope to clear the airway
(e) ventilate with positive resuscitator

5.34 A male was injured when a gas stove exploded in his face. He is conscious but has blistering around the mouth, nares, and left cheek. In addition to his obvious surface trauma, you should suspect that he might also have
(a) carbon monoxide poisoning
(b) respiratory burns
(c) cerebral edema
(d) cardiac arrhythmias
(e) hypertension

5.35 Which of the following are most likely to be included in the treatment of pulmonary edema:
(a) morphine, sodium bicarbonate, and calcium chloride
(b) Demerol, Isuprel, and Lanoxin
(c) Lanoxin, Lasix, and Isuprel
(d) Lasix, morphine, and Aminophylline
(e) Aminophylline, Intropin, and sodium bicarbonate

5.36 Initial action in an unconscious apneic patient with suspected upper airway obstruction should be
(a) position the head and attempt to ventilate
(b) examine the mouth and oropharynx

(c) visualize the obstruction with a laryngoscope
(d) insert EOA
(e) perform cricothyrotomy

5.37 A patient who exhibits acute respiratory distress, crowing, stridor, tracheal indrawing, and use of accessory muscles of respiration should be suspected of having
(a) pneumothorax
(b) pneumonia
(c) tension pneumothorax
(d) emphysema
(e) upper airway obstruction

5.38 Which of the following disorders should *not* receive high flow oxygen:
(a) asthma
(b) myocardial infarction
(c) trauma
(d) chronic bronchitis
(e) pleurisy

5.39 In which of the following circumstances is cricothyrotomy *most* likely to be indicated:
(a) allergic reaction
(b) status asthmaticus
(c) respiratory arrest following aspiration
(d) complete airway obstruction caused by epiglottitis
(e) respiratory arrest following respiratory burns

5.40 Which of the following would suggest that the EOA was positioned in the trachea:
(a) absence of breath sounds on one or both sides
(b) absence of gag reflex
(c) rales in the bases of one or both lungs
(d) good ventilation of both lungs
(e) coughing

5.41 Ammonia ampules should be used with caution in COPD patients because they may precipitate
(a) syncope
(b) bronchospasm
(c) hypotension
(d) respiratory depression
(e) vomiting

5.42 Which of the following commonly provides the respiratory drive in patients with COPD:
(a) changes in pH
(b) changes in tidal volume
(c) low serum oxygen level

(d) high serum carbon dioxide level
(e) high O_2 and CO_2 levels

5.43 A male is having substernal pain and you suspect that he is having an MI. He tells you that he has chronic emphysema. Despite being given oxygen at 4 l per minute he continues to be increasingly cyanotic. You should expect to
(a) have him breathe into a paper bag
(b) intubate him and ventilate with positive pressure
(c) give Aminophylline and sodium bicarbonate and reduce oxygen flow rate
(d) increase oxygen flow rate and be prepared to ventilate
(e) reduce the amount of oxygen even further but compensate by increasing IV flow rate

5.44 Aminophylline should be administered
(a) IV drip mixed with 500 ml 5 percent D/W
(b) deep IM into a major muscle mass
(c) IV push directly into the vein
(d) rapidly into the IV line
(e) slowly via IV Volutrol

5.45 A classic sign of upper airway obstruction is
(a) vomiting or repeated swallowing
(b) inspiratory stridor
(c) wheezing
(d) slow respiratory rate
(e) Kussmaul breathing

5.46 How would you modify your procedure for applying rotating tourniquets on a patient with an IV in one extremity:
(a) apply three tourniquets and don't rotate them
(b) apply two tourniquets and rotate them on unaffected limbs
(c) apply three tourniquets and rotate them without regard to the IV
(d) apply four tourniquets and don't rotate them
(e) apply tourniquets only to legs and remove after 15 minutes

5.47 Signs of pulmonary edema include all of the following *except*
(a) apprehension
(b) decreased level of consciousness
(c) frothy sputum
(d) bradycardia
(e) distended neck veins

5.48 Which of the following is the *incorrect* technique for nasotracheal suctioning:
(a) give oxygen before and after suctioning
(b) lubricate tip of the catheter
(c) insert catheter to the carina

(d) if you meet resistance, apply firm pressure until the obstruction is passed
(e) apply suction only when withdrawing the catheter, not while inserting it

5.49 Which of the following is *not* true about rotating tourniquets:
(a) they are used to treat pulmonary edema
(b) they are applied to three of four extremities
(c) they are applied so that arterial flow is not impaired
(d) they are rotated at regular intervals
(e) they can all be removed at one time

ANSWER KEY

5.1 b	**5.13** e	**5.25** e	**5.37** e
5.2 d	**5.14** c	**5.26** a	**5.38** d
5.3 a	**5.15** b	**5.27** d	**5.39** d
5.4 b	**5.16** b	**5.28** b	**5.40** a
5.5 d	**5.17** b	**5.29** c	**5.41** b
5.6 a	**5.18** d	**5.30** d	**5.42** c
5.7 a	**5.19** d	**5.31** e	**5.43** d
5.8 b	**5.20** b	**5.32** d	**5.44** e
5.9 e	**5.21** a	**5.33** a	**5.45** b
5.10 b	**5.22** a	**5.34** b	**5.46** b
5.11 b	**5.23** b	**5.35** d	**5.47** d
5.12 c	**5.24** a	**5.36** a	**5.48** d
			5.49 e

6

CARDIOVASCULAR EMERGENCIES

CASE STUDY 6A: MR. J. TUTTLE

Your paramedic unit responds to a call for a man "not breathing" at a local restaurant. A nearby fire department engine is simultaneously dispatched to the scene and arrives within three minutes. When you and your partner arrive, CPR is already in progress. Your patient is a male in his late 50s, who weighs approximately 220 pounds. His skin is warm, dry, and slightly cyanotic. Pupils are dilated but respond very sluggishly to light. A quick check through the defibrillator paddles shows fine ventricular fibrillation on the monitor.

Prior to defibrillating, the patient medic should quickly

1. intubate the patient
2. take over ventilation of the patient
3. ensure effectiveness of CPR
4. start an IV line

Although defibrillation is the obvious treatment of choice, the effectiveness of CPR is critical to all subsequent treatment. It is unwise to assume, when CPR is already in progress, that it is being performed effectively. Therefore, it is imperative that the paramedic team immediately assess the effectiveness of both ventilation (adequate chest expansion and breath sounds) and circulation (palpable pulses with each chest compression).

After assessing the effectiveness of CPR, your partner defibrillates once, and the patient goes into asystole. Meanwhile, you establish communication with the hospital. Your initial report is brief. Immediately you are instructed to insert an endotracheal tube and establish an IV line. After receiving the anticipated orders, you switch to continuous EKG telemetry. The airway is inserted without difficulty, and both the patient's arms are bared for possible IV sites. After one unsuccessful attempt at an antecubital IV, the decision is made to attempt an external jugular line. An IV cannula is selected with a syringe attached and, with CPR still in progress, your partner makes a perfect stick.

A possible complication of the external jugular IV site is

1. pneumothorax
2. laceration of a carotid artery
3. air embolus
4. all of the above

An external jugular IV is a reasonable choice when more conventional peripheral sites are unavailable. It is, however, not without risk for the patient; each choice is a potential hazard with this technique. Though relatively superficial, the external jugular vein also lies close to the carotid arteries; unsuccessful placement of a cannula may penetrate these vessels or enter the pleural cavity.

With the IV established and well taped in place, you are instructed to give 1 mg epinephrine 1:10,000. After about one minute the patient's rhythm changes to a coarse ventricular fibrillation. The hospital also notes the change in rhythm and suggests defibrillation with full output discharge. Your partner has already put gel on the paddles and waits as the defibrillator charges. CPR is stopped, and the patient's body lurches characteristically as the current is delivered. The monitor continues to show ventricular fibrillation. A second defibrillation is given, but this time a slow ventricular rhythm results. There is a weak, palpable pulse present at a rate of 30. The monitor shows complete heart block (CHB) with an underlying junctional focus.

Of the following drugs, which will be used initially for treating this arrhythmia (CHB):

1. Isuprel, 1–2 mg in 5 percent D/W
2. Inderal, 1–4 mg IV
3. Lidocaine, 100 mg IV
4. atropine, 0.5–1 mg IV

Heart blocks result from insult to the heart's conduction system (infarction, contusion, etc.). Atropine is effective in treating heart blocks by suppressing parasympathetic tone and enhancing conduction through the AV junction. Therefore, ventricular depolarization, which comes from a junctional focus, should respond to atropine.

Atropine, 1 mg IV push, is ordered. Following the atropine, Lidocaine is also to be given, 100 mg IV. As the patient's pulse slowly increases, chest compressions are stopped, and the gurney is brought in. The patient is breathing on his own at a rate of 8, so you continue to assist ventilations. Transport of this patient to the emergency room is started.

En route with a 10 minute ETA, you pick up the radio handset to update the hospital on your patient's current status. The voice transmission from the hospital, however, comes back very garbled and broken. As you quickly troubleshoot your radio, everything seems to be in order. A freshly charged battery is quickly installed, but this offers no improvement. (A broken antenna lead later proves to be the culprit.) Your partner directs your attention to the monitor, which shows frequent ventricular ectopics. Suddenly the patient seizes and goes into ventricular fibrillation.

Of the following choices which would you now elect to do:

1. push another 50 mg of Lidocaine
2. defibrillate immediately
3. give an additional amp of sodium bicarbonate
4. give Diazepam for the seizure

Current protocols for advanced cardiac life-support advocate precordial thump and immediate defibrillation as the treatment of choice when cardiac arrest due to ventricular fibrillation is monitored. CPR should also be initiated at once. Administration of drugs in the absence of direct voice contact with the hospital is not approved in some EMS programs. Under such circumstances, where there are no standing orders, the paramedic is ethically obligated to perform within the legal limits of that system's guidelines.

You deliver a precordial thump and begin to administer CPR as your partner charges the defibrillator. Within a few seconds your partner places the paddles on the patient's chest and, when you have pulled away, your partner delivers the countershock. The rhythm again converts to a complete heart block but, because the pulse is extremely bradycardic, you continue CPR. The ambulance pulls in front of the ED entrance, and the gurney is wheeled inside. Your partner takes over CPR, while you brief the doctor on the patient's condition. The decision is made to insert a transvenous pacemaker in order to stabilize the patient's rhythm. The antecubital site is carefully prepped, and the catheter is slowly introduced until the pacemaker blip on the monitor indicates that it is effectively placed. Your patient is transferred to the coronary care unit (CCU), where he later receives a permanent pacemaker.

Cardiac arrest is almost commonplace for most prehospital care teams. Treatment routinely follows established protocols, but even so the survival rate is dishearteningly low. Complicating factors such as elapsed time of arrest prior to CPR, aspiration after regurgitation, and difficulties encountered while moving the patient to the ambulance contribute heavily to these grim statistics. Success, however, may be enhanced by effective CPR, careful airway management by means of esophageal or endotracheal intubation, and prompt and accurate administration of IV drugs.

Your patient survives his cardiac arrest and is a "save," owing in large part to competent, advanced prehospital care.

CASE STUDY 6B: MR. R. MORGAN

An emergency telephone call is made to the emergency services dispatch center in your city via 911. The frantic woman caller asks for an ambulance to help her husband, who is having a lot of trouble breathing. It is 11 o'clock in the evening. Calmly and quickly the dispatcher obtains the necessary information and reassures the distressed woman that paramedics will be there in a few minutes. Within moments your paramedic rescue unit and a fire department engine company are notified to respond.

When you and your partner arrive at the modest mobile home, you are met at the door by a woman in her 60s, who leads you into the living room where her husband is sitting on an overstuffed chair. He also appears to be in his late 60s, is markedly short of breath, and is quite pale and diaphoretic. Quickly your partner obtains pertinent medical history from the wife while you put the patient on oxygen at 6 l by mask. Even before you put the stethoscope to your ears to auscultate lung sounds, you note audible respiratory congestion sounds on both inspiration and expiration. Breath sounds confirm coarse bilateral rales, especially on inspiration.

The next most logical step in your physical exam should be to

1. look for distended neck veins
2. perform a thorough neurological exam
3. check the pulse and monitor the EKG
4. immediately start an IV

Following an assessment of the airway and breathing should come a check of the pulse (both rate and quality) and EKG rhythm. Although this patient is obviously in severe distress, the urgency to perform a rapid physical exam should never rule out the necessity of following the ABCs.

The patient's radial pulse is 130 and weak. Owing to excessive skin moisture, you carefully wipe his chest and apply the electrode pads. Your monitor shows a sinus tachycardia. Because your patient is very dyspneic and apprehensive, you ask him short and concise questions. He does have a history of heart problems and normally gets short of breath upon exertion. Tonight he became short of breath about 45 minutes after retiring to bed. He is taking Lanoxin and Lasix daily. Completing your physical exam, you find that your patient has marked distention of his jugular veins. His respirations are 36 and labored, blood pressure is 160/100. He is having no chest pain at this time. The engine company has just arrived on the scene.

After contacting the base station, which of the following choices would not be indicated for this patient:

1. morphine, 2–15 mg IV
2. antishock trousers
3. rotating tourniquets
4. Furosemide, 20–40 mg IV

Treatment of pulmonary edema due to congestive heart failure is based upon reducing the cardiac workload by decreasing right heart return. Morphine eases respiratory effort and along with rotating tourniquets causes venous pooling in the peripheral vasculature. Furosemide (Lasix) is a potent diuretic and thus reduces circulating volume. Antishock trousers are absolutely contraindicated, because this device would obviously increase right heart return.

Upon initial radio contact with the hospital, your partner describes the patient's current status. You are requested to apply rotating tourniquets and start an IV with D_5W to keep open. Initially, you place the tourniquets on all four extremities, as high as possible, and prepare to start the IV in the patient's forearm. Your partner makes a note of the time and informs the hospital that the tourniquet on that arm is removed, leaving three extremities with occluded venous return. With no history of COPD, you increase the oxygen to 10 l, as you note the patient has some cyanosis. A recheck of vital signs shows that the pulse is 132, respirations remain 36 and extremely labored, and BP is 160/108. Your partner relays the updated vital signs and receives an order for morphine sulfate, 6 mg slow IV. As you slowly administer the morphine, you glance at the monitor, which shows atrial fibrillation.

Which of the following statements about this arrhythmia is true:

1. it should be defibrillated immediately
2. it is rarely encountered in the field
3. it is easily confused with V fib
4. it has no discernible P waves

Atrial fibrillation is normally a benign arrhythmia, which requires no field treatment unless the rate is excessive. It is easily identifiable by a grossly irregular R-R interval and no indistinguishable P waves.

With 6 mg of MS on board, you note that the patient is less anxious and seems to have less labored respiratory effort. You reauscultate breath sounds and still hear rales throughout the base of each lung; however, you believe that there is some improvement. The hospital orders 40 mg Lasix IV to start and requests that you transport as soon as possible. A firefighter brings in the gurney, and the patient is moved onto it.

Which of the following positions is most appropriate for this patient:

1. Trendelenberg (head down)
2. sitting upright
3. right lateral decubitus (lying on right side)
4. supine with a pillow

Any conscious patient with dyspnea will be most comfortable in an upright sitting position. In patients with pulmonary edema, reclining positions allow venous return from the lower body, which increases right heart return. In addition, these positions restrict ventilatory effort when abdominal organs press up against the diaphragm.

Just prior to transport, you administer the Lasix IV push as ordered. Vital signs are pulse 120 and irregular, respirations 28 and slightly labored, and blood pressure 126/90. Rales are diminished but still present bilaterally. Upon arrival at the hospital, your patient seems to have stabilized. The emergency room doctor congratulates you and your partner along with the radio nurse for your rapid assessment and treatment.

Discussion

Patients with acute respiratory emergencies have the potential to deteriorate very rapidly. This is especially true in the case of a CHF patient with pulmonary edema. Though their primary problem is cardiac in nature, respiratory involvement ensues when poor left ventricular ejection causes engorgement of the pulmonary vasculature. Fluid is forced into the alveoli, leading to hypoxia and poor perfusion. Treatment in the prehospital phase is aimed at decreasing the cardiac workload to improve pump efficiency and increasing blood oxygen saturation. In severe cases, positive pressure ventilation with an oxygen-powered resuscitator and mask may be helpful to force fluid out the alveoli to improve the ventilatory effort.

After respiratory therapy treatment in the ED, your patient is admitted in good condition to the hospital for three days and then released.

CASE STUDY 6C: MR. E. GORDON

It has been a quiet shift for your normally busy station on this winter's day. Almost inevitably, however, the station alarm sounds just as you are sitting down to an evening meal.

"Medic six, engine four, respond to a possible heart attack in the restaurant, 326 East Brougham Avenue."

Your partner quickly disconnects the electrical cord supplying power to the battery chargers of your various biomedical equipment. You pull the two-year-old, type III ambulance into the street. Within minutes you arrive in front of the popular downtown restaurant.

Inside you find a man in his late 60s who complains of severe epigastric pain. His skin is pale and moist, and he appears quite anxious. His EKG shows normal sinus rhythm at a rate of 92, and his blood pressure is 168/110. The patient has no breathing difficulty, and he does not have any previous cardiac history.

Which is the most useful to further determine the possible cause of this patient's condition:

1. bilateral blood pressures
2. palpation of the abdomen
3. further investigation of the chief complaint
4. no further information is required

The patient information presented thus far offers few clues that might differentiate between several possible causes for the pain. Thus, further investigation of the chief complaint is definitely indicated. Palpation of the abdomen as well as taking bilateral blood pressures should be performed later as part of the physical exam.

Upon more questioning the patient tells you that his pain came on suddenly as he was eating. He describes it as a sharp, excruciating pain just below the xiphoid that now has radiated into his back and upper abdomen. Breath sounds are clear, pulses are equal, and blood pressures are the same bilaterally. The abdomen is soft but tender to palpation in both upper quadrants. The patient previously has had no nausea or vomiting, and his stools are normal. The rest of the exam is unremarkable, and hypertension is the only medical problem for which he is being treated. As you put the patient on oxygen by cannula, your partner contacts the hospital for an initial IV order.

The *least* likely cause for the patient's symptoms is

1. acute pancreatitis
2. perforated duodenal ulcer

3. dissecting aortic aneurysm
4. none of the above

Though somewhat misleading, this question should remind you that there are often several pathologic dysfunctions that might be present with nearly identical symptoms. As yet, none of these diagnoses can safely be ruled out. It is important that the prehospital care team treat cautiously in such cases unless arrhythmias, hypotension, or other signs of rapid deterioration are observed.

The hospital requests that an IV line be established with lactated Ringer's, to infuse at 200 cc per hour. Cardiac monitoring and updated vital signs are to be reported en route. Before you start the IV, however, your patient suddenly becomes unresponsive. The EKG monitor displays a junctional tachycardia, and, although he continues to breath adequately on his own, the pulse is weakly palpable. His blood pressure is 40/0.

Immediate intervention for this patient would *not* include

1. Intropin (dopamine) IV
2. antishock trousers
3. high flow oxygen by mask
4. central venous line

The rapid onset of shock in this patient probably indicates a catastrophic cardiac or vascular emergency has occurred. Treatment must now be aggressive in order to reverse both hypotension and hypoxia and would include antishock trousers, oxygen by mask, and a central venous line (if permitted under local protocols). Dopamine is an appropriate pharmacologic agent in cases of cardiogenic or septisemic shock; however, it should not be utilized for suspected hypovolemia until adequate volume replacement has been accomplished.

While your partner fits an oxygen mask to the patient's face, you slide the antishock trousers underneath the patient's legs.

Since your EMS program authorizes a central venous line when peripheral sites are unavailable, you carefully prep the proper site over the internal jugular vein with Betadine. After puncturing the skin with the large bore needle, you angle the cannula into the vein. The tubing is attached, and the catheter is securely taped in place. The blood pressure is now 80/40, and the patient moans incoherently. A second IV bag is hung as you squeeze the first liter, forcibly infusing the fluid as quickly as possible. Soon you are at the hospital, and scrub-suited emergency room staff open the ambulance's back door to assist you. A surgical team has been notified, and the OR is ready. A stat type and crossmatch for blood has been ordered and is quickly drawn by an experienced lab technician. Within three minutes after arriving at the hospital your patient is in surgery where a ruptured abdominal aortic aneurysm is discovered and repaired.

Discussion

Aneurysms can occur within the wall of any blood vessel. In some cases they may be benign and remain undiscovered. In other cases, however, they may enlarge, leak, or rupture with often lethal results. Fatal cerebrovascular accidents are frequently attributed to this cause.

An aneurysm in the aorta may also rupture with a rapid loss of blood. More often, however, the patient may experience a dissecting aneurysm as high intra-arterial pressure causes a separation of vascular tissue in the wall of the vessel. Depending upon its location in the aorta, this type of aneurysm may produce unequal bilateral pulses of the upper or lower extremities or unequal blood pressure values as blood flow is impeded by the dissection. These injuries are usually very painful and may be described by the patient as a "ripping" or "tearing" pain that radiates through to the back.

Treatment is supportive in most cases, paying close attention to vital signs. Deterioration of the patient's condition warrants aggressive treatment and immediate transport to the nearest surgical facility.

Your patient is discharged after three weeks in surgical intensive care and is able to return to his normal active lifestyle after recuperating fully. Your prompt and competent actions have saved his life.

CASES STUDY 6D: MR. A. MENDOZA

"Medic 3, respond with the fire department to a traffic accident, vehicle reported into a building." Within moments you and your partner are en route to the downtown location. Three blocks away from the scene, traffic is tightly congested as afternoon rush hour, combined with curious onlookers, creates a nearly impassable situation. Police are directing cars onto side streets, and soon you are able to pull up to the accident. Water from a sheared-off hydrant spews 30 feet into the air. There seems to be a single vehicle involved that is sitting on its roof half way into a multi-story office building. There is severe damage to the front end of the car; one patient is visible in the front seat.

Which would not be among your immediate considerations in this case:

1. determining if any other patients are involved
2. assessing the potential building collapse
3. establishing radio contact with the hospital
4. gaining access to the patient

There are always several determinations that are made soon after arriving at an accident such as this one. The least immediate priority in this case, however, is establishing communication with the hospital, because very little information is yet known.

The vehicle has crashed through a large window, but there is little other observable damage to the building. The car itself is in a stable position, and there are no other people injured because office workers have left for the day.

Crawling through the shattered rear window of the sedan, you find the patient, a male in his late 30s, lying on his back between the front seat and the headliner. He is conscious. His breathing seems to be adequate, and his pulse is 120. He complains of pain in the back of his neck, his right shoulder, and chest. His skin is warm, dry, and pale. Blood pressure is weakly palpable at 110.

In what order would you treat this patient:

1. immobilize spine, IV, oxygen, monitor, extricate
2. immobilize spine, extricate, oxygen, monitor, IV
3. extricate, IV, oxygen, monitor, transport
4. immobilize spine, extricate, transport immediately

Careful immobilization of the spine is obviously indicated prior to moving this patient with oxygen, IV, and monitor attached. These therapies are best performed after the patient is removed from the vehicle. One exception to this principle is when extrication is prolonged, and immediate treatment is indicated.

Since space inside the overturned vehicle is limited, you remain inside with the patient. Quickly, you confer with your partner, who is looking in the passenger door window. Your plan is to place a cervical collar on the patient, slide him onto a backboard and then out through the passenger door, which must be forced open. Fire department personnel are standing by to aid in the rescue effort. A hydraulic spreader is set up to pry open the jammed door. Meanwhile, the patient continues to complain of chest pain and now some shortness of breath. Time is beginning to work against you. Looking up, you also notice something else for the first time: The steering wheel has been crushed into the dashboard.

Fortunately, you are able to slide the patient onto the backboard and out the door opened by the firefighters. The patient is quickly carried to the waiting gurney and into the ambulance. Vital signs now show his pulse is 130, blood pressure is 90/80, and respirations are 32. Breath sounds are clear bilaterally.

In addition to being hypotensive, his blood pressure also indicates a

1. paradoxial pulse
2. mediastinal shift

3. compensatory pause
4. narrow pulse pressure

The differential between the systolic and diastolic pressures is known as the pulse pressure. This patient has a markedly narrow pulse pressure, which is consistent with a developing tension pneumothorax, hemothorax, or cardiac tamponade.

Upon examination of the patient, you discover a large contusion on the anterior chest. The chest wall seems to be intact and has equal expansion with each inspiratory effort. There are also deformity in his right distal clavical and minor facial lacerations. You put him on oxygen at 8 l/min by mask and hook up the chest leads for the monitor. The rhythm is sinus tachycardia with occasional premature ventricular contractions. The hospital orders an IV and stat transport. The patient's skin is now pale, cool, and moist, and he is increasingly anxious. You decide to transport now and try for the IV en route to the hospital. A recheck of breath sounds still shows them to be clear in all fields. Heart sounds are present but barely audible in the back of the ambulance.

Upon arrival at the hospital, the patient becomes very restless and confused. He complains of severe chest pain. The emergency room physician orders stat portable X-rays of the chest and lateral cervical spine, as well as arterial blood gases. Vital signs are now pulse 136, blood pressure 82/64, and respirations 40. The doctor also auscultates the chest thoroughly and determines that the patient probably has a cardiac tamponade. A chest tray is quickly set up for a pericardiocentesis, and the physician selects a 20 cc syringe with a four-inch intracardiac needle. The skin is prepped just below the left costal margin, and the doctor carefully inserts the needle just left of the xiphoid process. After the needle is advanced about three inches, the syringe suddenly begins to fill with blood. A total of 40 cc is drawn out, by using a second syringe. Vital signs begin to improve dramatically, and the patient is monitored closely.

Discussion

Cardiac tamponade is not seen frequently by most paramedics. Because definitive therapy, pericardiocentesis, is rarely medically or legally sanctioned in the field, treatment must be aimed at immediate transport. A patient with cardiac tamponade can and will continue to deteriorate because cardiac output is diminished with each beat. IV fluids are contraindicated because ensuing shock is cardiogenic in nature.

Signs and symptoms of cardiac tamponade include tachycardia, neck vein distension, muffled heart sounds, cyanosis, hypotension, and severe shock. Treatment should include high flow oxygen, cardiac monitor, and an intravenous line TKO. Under no circumstances should transport be delayed if tamponade is suspected.

Owing in part to the rapid diagnosis of his medical emergency, your patient survives and recovers from his injuries. He is discharged home after three weeks in the hospital's intensive care unit.

RELATED ASSESSMENT QUESTIONS

6.1 A pulsating abdominal mass is suggestive of
(a) ruptured spleen
(b) appendicitis
(c) arrhythmias
(d) aneurysm
(e) hypertension

6.2 Valsalva's maneuver is performed to
(a) improve conduction through the AV node
(b) reduce ventricular irritability
(c) slow the heart rate
(d) dilate the coronary arteries
(e) enhance the sinus node

6.3 Which of the following is the most appropriate parameter to monitor during Aramine administration:
(a) EKG
(b) respirations
(c) deep tendon reflexes
(d) blood pressure
(e) pulse

6.4 Which of the following is *not* an acceptable site for an intracardiac injection in an adult:
(a) 4th intercostal space, 2 cm left of sternum
(b) 4th intercostal space, midaxillary line
(c) immediately below and left of xiphoid process
(d) 5th intercostal space, 2 cm left of sternum
(e) all are acceptable sites

6.5 Morphine sulfate is contraindicated in all of the following *except*
(a) respiratory depression
(b) isolated head injury
(c) acute abdominal pain
(d) pulmonary edema
(e) hypotension

6.6 The most common cause of death within the first few hours of a myocardial infarction is
(a) ventricular failure
(b) shock

(c) arrhythmia
(d) coronary occlusion
(e) ruptured aneurysm

6.7 Which of the following is the most appropriate initial w/s setting for defibrillating ventricular fibrillation in an adult:
(a) 200 w/s
(b) 400 w/s
(c) 1 w/s per kg
(d) 20–25 w/s per kg
(e) 5–6 w/s per kg

6.8 The dosage of Levophed when mixed in 250–500 ml of 5 percent D/W is
(a) 0.4 mg, titrated to pulse
(b) 100–200 mg, run at 20–40 gtt per min
(c) 1–2 gm, titrated to blood pressure
(d) 4–8 mg, titrated to blood pressure
(e) 15–20 mg, not to exceed 5 micrograms per min

6.9 To treat a patient in cardiogenic shock, you would use
(a) morphine and epinephrine
(b) dopamine and oxygen
(c) IV fluids and Aminophylline
(d) Lidocaine and antishock trousers
(e) Lasix and Trendelenberg position

6.10 You would consider giving Lidocaine prophylactically to all patients who
(a) are sensitive to narcotics and other analgesics
(b) are experiencing chest pain consistent with MI
(c) are receiving vasopressors
(d) might be a candidate for cardioversion
(e) have a heart rate greater than 150 beats per minute

6.11 The dosage range for Lasix is
(a) 1–2 gm
(b) 10–20 mEq
(c) 20–80 mg
(d) 250–500 ml
(e) 25–50 gr

6.12 Which of the following is *most* likely to be associated with congestive heart failure:
(a) internal bleeding
(b) cerebral emboli
(c) thrombophlebitis
(d) pneumothorax
(e) pulmonary edema

6.13 Which of the following is the *least* characteristic of congestive heart failure:
(a) distended neck veins
(b) difficulty in breathing
(c) hemoptysis
(d) cyanosis
(e) tachycardia

6.14 Your patient is allergic to sulfonamides. This warns you to use caution if you need to administer
(a) Lasix
(b) morphine
(c) Physostigmine
(d) Isuprel
(e) Levophed

6.15 The patient who complains of crushing chest pain and is having PVCs most likely requires
(a) nitroglycerine and Isuprel
(b) Lidocaine and atropine
(c) sodium bicarbonate and nitroglycerine
(d) morphine and Lidocaine
(e) atropine and morphine

6.16 It is not a good idea to determine the pulse rate from the monitor since it
(a) tells you about the electrical activity but not about mechanical activity
(b) is usually about 20 beats per minute too fast
(c) is distorted by telemetry
(d) reflects activity of the upper chambers of the heart, but not the ventricles
(e) none of the above; it is perfectly acceptable to count the pulse by checking the monitor

6.17 Which of the following is *least* likely to be a complication of acute MI:
(a) hypotension
(b) laryngospasm
(c) arrhythmias
(d) sudden death
(e) pulmonary edema

6.18 When preparing to defibrillate a patient found in ventricular fibrillation, you should do all of the following *except*
(a) order all personnel to "stand clear"
(b) check pulses and lead wires
(c) ensure the synchronization button is on

(d) give sodium bicarbonate and epinephrine
(e) perform cardiopulmonary resuscitation

6.19 Which of the following is *not* a typical location of the chest pain associated with MI and thus could suggest something else:
(a) substernal
(b) lower abdomen
(c) left or right arm
(d) epigastric
(e) neck, jaw, and/or teeth

6.20 Ventricular irritability in the presence of myocardial infarction is
(a) to be expected and not a cause for alarm
(b) a precursor to respiratory involvement
(c) very dangerous and should be treated
(d) highly unlikely if oxygen is administered
(e) only treated if it causes symptoms

6.21 Which of the following features characteristically informs you that nitroglycerine is still fresh and, if absent, suggests that the drug is outdated:
(a) blood pressure rises
(b) patient gets drowsy
(c) bottle "whooshes" when opened
(d) skeletal muscles quiver momentarily
(e) pill tastes bitter

6.22 Which of the following statements best explains the process of defibrillating a patient who has a pacemaker implanted in the chest:
(a) this patient can't be defibrillated because it would cause severe myocardial damage
(b) defibrillation will damage the pacemaker and hence should not be performed
(c) the patient can be defibrillated, but the pacemaker must first be turned off with a magnet
(d) defibrillation will not hurt the pacemaker at all and should be performed without concern for the pacemaker
(e) defibrillation will damage the pacemaker and probably the myocardium, but must be performed anyway

6.23 Cardiac arrest is best identified by assessing
(a) respirations and pulses
(b) pupils and respirations
(c) pupils and EKG
(d) EKG and pulses
(e) EKG and respirations

6.24 An *early* sign of Lidocaine toxicity is
(a) seizure activity
(b) irritability and apprehension
(c) asystole or ventricular standstill
(d) hypertension
(e) Cheyne-Stokes respirations

6.25 The dosage of nitroglycerine is
(a) 200 gr every 5 minutes times 3
(b) 0.4 mg, repeated if needed
(c) 5 mg initially, followed by 2 mg in 10 minutes
(d) 25 mg once only
(e) 0.5 gr, may repeat once

6.26 Which of the following is the *most* likely indication for the use of nitroglycerine:
(a) hypotension
(b) angina pectoris
(c) migraine headache
(d) cardiogenic shock
(e) coma of unknown origin

6.27 Atropine toxicity is characterized by all of the following *except*
(a) dry mouth
(b) pupil dilatation
(c) cold, clammy skin
(d) hallucinations
(e) depressed level of consciousness

6.28 In a middle-age patient who complains of indigestion and difficulty in breathing, you should
(a) allow the EMT ambulance to transport
(b) have the patient see a private physician
(c) give oxygen, monitor the EKG, and start an IV
(d) monitor the EKG, give dopamine, and transport "red light and siren"
(e) give oxygen and bicarbonate of soda and transport

6.29 Which of the following are indications for the use of atropine:
(a) hypotension and ventricular irritability
(b) bradycardia and hypovolemia
(c) hypertension and heart blocks
(d) bradycardia and organophosphate poisoning
(e) tachyarrhythmias and Valium overdose

6.30 If cardioversion must be performed on a conscious patient, you should first
(a) restrain the patient
(b) raise the w/s setting

(c) give Lidocaine to numb the area
(d) give Valium to sedate the patient
(e) give morphine for the pain

6.31 The dosage of calcium chloride is
(a) 1–2 gm
(b) 4–8 mg
(c) 50–100 mg
(d) 250–500 mg
(e) 50 mEq

6.32 You have been ordered to administer epinephrine prior to defibrillating a patient in ventricular fibrillation. The most appropriate dosage for this situation is
(a) 0.3 mg 1:1,000 SC
(b) 0.5–1 mg 1:1,000 IM
(c) 0.5–1 mg 1:10,000 IV
(d) 5–10 mg 1:10,000 IV
(e) 5–10 mg 1:1,000 IV

6.33 Which of the following would *most* likely be included in the management of any patient in cardiac arrest:
(a) EKG, epinephrine, IV, and oxygen at 4 l/min
(b) high flow oxygen, IV, EKG, and vasopressors
(c) CPR, dopamine, and prompt transport
(d) IV, intubation, antishock trousers, and Narcan
(e) CPR, IV, EKG, and sodium bicarbonate

6.34 The correct dosage of Isuprel when mixed in 500 ml of 5 percent D/W is
(a) 1–2 mg
(b) 2–5 mg
(c) 5–10 mg
(d) 25–50 mg
(e) 100–250 mg

6.35 Which of the following drugs is *most* likely to produce a cumulative effect when given with Isuprel:
(a) epinephrine
(b) Valium
(c) sodium bicarbonate
(d) Lidocaine
(e) calcium chloride

6.36 The expected duration of Lidocaine is
(a) less than 5 minutes
(b) 10 to 20 minutes
(c) 30 minutes to 1 hour

(d) 1 to 4 hours
(e) 8 to 12 hours

6.37 An initial bolus of Lidocaine should always be followed by
(a) atropine IV push
(b) vasopressors
(c) defibrillation
(d) additional Lidocaine by bolus or drip
(e) sodium bicarbonate IV push or drip

6.38 Which of the following is the most appropriate field treatment of cardiogenic shock:
(a) IV fluid replacement, oxygen, and morphine
(b) oxygen, antishock trousers, and IV Ringer's lactate
(c) dopamine, IV TKO, and oxygen
(d) IV TKO, shock position, and oxygen
(e) shock position, IV fluid replacement, and dopamine

6.39 Nitroglycerine is used for anginal pain because it
(a) anesthetizes the myocardium
(b) reduces cardiac workload
(c) slows the heart rate
(d) increases the oxygen-carrying capacity of the blood
(e) interrupts the pain sensations at the synapse

6.40 Which of the following is the most likely therapy for a patient who has cardiac tamponade and is rapidly deteriorating despite your supportive therapy:
(a) pericardiocentesis
(b) needle thoracostomy
(c) antishock trousers
(d) defibrillation
(e) cardiac pacemaker

6.41 The most common cause of death in a patient with an MI is
(a) cardiogenic shock
(b) arrhythmias
(c) hypertension
(d) renal failure
(e) pulmonary embolus

6.42 When Inderal is given to break a supraventricular tachycardia, the appropriate dosage and route are
(a) 8 mg in 500 ml 5 percent D/W, titrated to B/P
(b) 1 gm IV Volutrol over 20 minutes
(c) 1–4 mg slow IV push, titrated to effect
(d) 0.5–1 mg in 500 ml 5 percent D/W, titrated to pulse
(e) 10 mg deep IM

6.43 When giving atropine IV push to increase heart rate, the initial dose should be
(a) 0.1–0.5 mg
(b) 0.5–1 mg
(c) 1–2 mg
(d) 2–5 mg
(e) 5–10 mg

6.44 Which of the following is your major concern when administering morphine sulfate:
(a) hypertension
(b) muscle tremors
(c) hallucinations
(d) parasthesia
(e) respiratory depression

6.45 Dopamine has an advantage over Aramine and Levophed in that it raises the blood pressure while
(a) increasing pulse and respiration
(b) reducing ventricular irritability
(c) perfusing vital organs
(d) reducing respiratory distress
(e) prolonging AV conduction

6.46 The intracardiac route is used
(a) during all cardiac arrests
(b) whenever epinephrine or calcium chloride is given
(c) when other routes are not immediately available
(d) as long as the patient does not have a pulse
(e) in adults but not in children

6.47 The dosage of Isuprel (1:5,000) is
(a) 5 mg direct IV push
(b) 250 mg IV Volutrol over 30 minutes
(c) 1 gm in 500 ml 5 percent D/W, titrated
(d) 50 mg deep IM
(e) 1–2 mg in 250–500 ml 5 percent D/W, titrated

6.48 The electrocardiogram is used to
(a) determine whether the heart is beating
(b) detect valvular dysfunction
(c) determine pulse rate
(d) evaluate electrical activity in the heart
(e) all of the above

6.49 Which of the following is appropriate for hypovolemic shock but *not* for cardiogenic shock:
(a) keep the patient warm
(b) give high flow oxygen

(c) monitor the EKG
(d) start an IV
(e) place in shock position

6.50 A primary concern during the administration of Levophed is prevention of infiltration, since it can
(a) reverse the effects of the drug
(b) cause cardiac arrhythmias
(c) interfere with the administration of other drugs
(d) cause tissue necrosis
(e) cause systemic infection

6.51 Which of the following statements does *not* pertain to the administration of morphine sulfate:
(a) it should be given in small increments
(b) it is contraindicated in head injuries
(c) it should be titrated to effect
(d) it has a maximum dosage range of 20 mg
(e) it can inhibit respirations

6.52 Which of the following is the most appropriate dosage/route for the administration of Aramine:
(a) 100 mg slow IV push
(b) 100–200 mg in 500 ml 5 percent D/W titrated to B/P
(c) 0.5 mg deep IM, repeatable in 2 minutes
(d) 0.5 mg in 250/500 ml 5 percent D/W, titrated to B/P
(e) 500 mg in 500 ml 5 percent D/W, titrated to pulse

6.53 Prior to performing carotid sinus massage, you should do all of the following *except*
(a) ensure that the carotid pulse is not diminished
(b) monitor the EKG
(c) have the patient perform Valsalva's maneuver
(d) establish a secure airway by intubating the trachea
(e) start an IV and give oxygen

6.54 Which of the following best describes the clinical symptoms associated with digitalis toxicity:
(a) GI disturbances, visual disturbances, and cardiac arrhythmias
(b) bronchoconstriction, hypotension, and tachycardia
(c) urticaria, respiratory distress, and shortening PRI
(d) nausea, inspiratory stridor, and nystagmus
(e) bigeminy, diplopia, and pedal edema

6.55 When Digoxin is used to convert a supraventricular tachycardia, the appropriate dosage and route are
(a) 1 mg sublingual, repeatable in 5 minutes
(b) 250 mg in 500 ml 5 percent D/W, titrated to effect
(c) 250 mg direct IV push

(d) 0.25–0.5 mg direct IV push
(e) 50–100 mg IV Volutrol over 20 minutes

6.56 Which of the following is *not* an indication for epinephrine:
(a) bradycardia
(b) ventricular fibrillation
(c) supraventricular tachycardia
(d) asthma
(e) anaphylaxis

6.57 When administering Aramine, it is essential that you
(a) first intubate the trachea
(b) recheck B/P every five minutes
(c) use a large bore cannula needle
(d) run Regitine simultaneously
(e) follow it with antishock trousers

6.58 Which of the following maneuvers will *not* help to improve contact between a monitoring electrode and the patient's skin:
(a) shaving excess hair
(b) applying conductive gel
(c) using a commercial ECG pad
(d) wetting the skin with water
(e) cleaning off dirt or dried blood

6.59 Cardioversion differs from defibrillation in that cardioversion is
(a) performed with anterior/posterior paddle placement
(b) tried after defibrillation has failed
(c) done without monitoring the EKG
(d) synchronized to avoid the T wave
(e) performed on conscious patients

6.60 Which of the following is a side effect of Levophed:
(a) sudden hypotension
(b) peripheral vasodilatation
(c) junctional tachyarrhythmias
(d) decreasing level of consciousness
(e) reflex bradycardia

6.61 Carotid sinus massage is reserved for use when a patient is experiencing a drop in cardiac output as a result of
(a) sustained tachyarrhythmia
(b) ventricular tachycardia
(c) ventricular fibrillation
(d) PVCs
(e) heart block

6.62 Which of the following statements about cardioversion is *not* true:
(a) it is synchronized to avoid hitting the T wave
(b) a conscious patient should be sedated before the procedure

(c) the watt/second setting is usually higher than for defibrillation
(d) paddle placement is the same as that for defibrillation
(e) the patient should be monitored during the procedure

6.63 Defibrillation is performed to terminate ventricular fibrillation. After the rhythm is converted, what drug might you give to prevent recurrence of this arrhythmia:
(a) Isuprel
(b) Aminophylline
(c) epinephrine
(d) Lidocaine
(e) calcium chloride

6.64 Calibrating an EKG tracing serves to
(a) standardize voltage
(b) adjust sweep speed
(c) determine monitoring lead
(d) make pacemaker blips more visible
(e) document time of radio transmission

6.65 After you attach your patient to the EKG monitor, you note quite a bit of 60-cycle interference. Which of the following maneuvers would be most likely to correct this problem:
(a) recheck electrode contact; improve contact if needed
(b) move the radio away from the monitor
(c) disconnect any electrical appliances in the vicinity
(d) switch to the telephone coupler
(e) change to another lead

6.66 You have an unconscious young man who apparently arrested following injection of some type of street drug. He is in ventricular fibrillation. Which of the following would *not* be included in your initial treatment of this patient:
(a) Isuprel
(b) defibrillation
(c) epinephrine
(d) Narcan
(e) sodium bicarbonate

6.67 The *most* reliable tools for diagnosing electromechanical dissociation are
(a) monitor and stethoscope
(b) B/P cuff and EKG calipers
(c) peripheral pulse and monitor
(d) monitor and reflex hammer
(e) B/P cuff and stethoscope

6.68 If your patient has a sustained tachyarrhythmia and is experiencing signs of dropping cardiac output, you would first try to slow the ventricular rate with vagotonic maneuvers but, if unsuccessful, might then try
- **(a)** Lidocaine or Brytellium
- **(b)** defibrillation
- **(c)** Inderal or Digoxin
- **(d)** hyperventilation
- **(e)** atropine or Isuprel

6.69 Which of the following maneuvers is *most* appropriate for treating a patient who is pulseless from ventricular tachycardia:
- **(a)** carotid sinus massage
- **(b)** Valsalva's maneuver
- **(c)** IV Lidocaine
- **(d)** defibrillation
- **(e)** cardioversion

6.70 Your patient has an internal pacemaker, but you cannot see the typical pacemaker spikes on the monitor. You should
- **(a)** defibrillate immediately
- **(b)** try another monitoring lead
- **(c)** use a magnet to increase pacemaker rate
- **(d)** transport immediately for a new battery
- **(e)** do nothing; the spikes should return on their own in a few minutes

6.71 An EKG pattern on a monitor can tell you all of the following *except*
- **(a)** which site is pacing the heart
- **(b)** at what rate the pacemaker is firing
- **(c)** whether the patient has an artificial pacemaker
- **(d)** whether the impulses are being conducted through the heart
- **(e)** whether the heart is pumping effectively

6.72 If your patient is in atrial fibrillation, you would expect to
- **(a)** defibrillate immediately
- **(b)** check for signs of CHF
- **(c)** give Lidocaine to slow rate
- **(d)** administer IV fluids
- **(e)** transport immediately for a pacemaker

6.73 Wenchebach differs from complete heart block in that CHB has
- **(a)** a regular R-R interval
- **(b)** a constant PRI
- **(c)** a faster rate
- **(d)** a normal QRS
- **(e)** upright P waves

6.74 If your monitor displays an EKG pattern with an inverted P wave, an inverted QRS complex, and an inverted T wave, you should first ensure that the patient has not experienced a sudden change in condition and then

(a) double-check lead placement
(b) disconnect the telephone coupler
(c) check for electrical interference such as lamps or electric blankets
(d) use your high-gain antenna
(e) switch to another lead, preferably MCL_1

6.75 The clinical manifestations (symptoms) of cardiac arrhythmias are usually a direct result of

(a) decreased peripheral resistance
(b) inadequate oxygenation
(c) drop in cardiac output
(d) low blood volume
(e) decreased level of consciousness

6.76 A patient in idioventricular rhythm would need

(a) a cardiac stimulant and CPR
(b) Lidocaine and defibrillation
(c) oxygen and carotid sinus massage
(d) Digoxin and oxygen
(e) a pacemaker and Lidocaine

6.77 The cardiac monitor can be used to diagnose electromechanical dissociation *only* if used in conjunction with

(a) IV Lidocaine
(b) cardioversion
(c) auscultation
(d) an artificial pacemaker
(e) a palpated pulse

CARDIAC ARRHYTHMIA SITUATIONS

Situation (refer to questions 6.78–6.82)

Your patient is female and is a 45-year-old director of a large publishing company. She has been experiencing a tightness in her chest for the last hour or two and is now having some nausea and difficulty breathing. Her only past illness was a hysterectomy 18 months ago. Her blood pressure is 124/86, respirations are 22. She seems concerned but is relatively calm and controlled. Her EKG shows the pattern seen in Figure 6–1.

6.78 This arrhythmia is

(a) complete heart block
(b) sinus arrhythmia
(c) Wenchebach (Mobitz I)

(d) sinus block
(e) second-degree heart block (Mobitz II)

6.79 This pattern can be serious, since it can lead to
(a) ventricular fibrillation
(b) sustained tachyarrhythmia
(c) congestive heart failure
(d) further blocks
(e) coronary insufficiency

6.80 Which of the following would you do to manage the patient's condition:
(a) give morphine and oxygen and consider dopamine
(b) start an IV, give oxygen and morphine, and monitor the EKG closely
(c) start an IV, give atropine, and consider morphine
(d) give atropine and Isuprel and transport promptly
(e) give IV fluids, give morphine, and monitor the EKG

6.81 During transport, the EKG changes to complete heart block with a rate of 36. Treatment of choice for this new pattern would be
(a) atropine and dopamine
(b) epinephrine and calcium chloride
(c) sodium bicarbonate and Lidocaine
(d) atropine and Isuprel
(e) Lidocaine and dopamine

6.82 The best treatment that you can offer the patient is
(a) a thorough assessment of lung sounds and a 12-lead EKG
(b) vasopressors and drugs to ease the pain
(c) drugs to suppress the ventricular focus
(d) rapid transport so that a pacemaker can be inserted
(e) antishock trousers and rapid transport

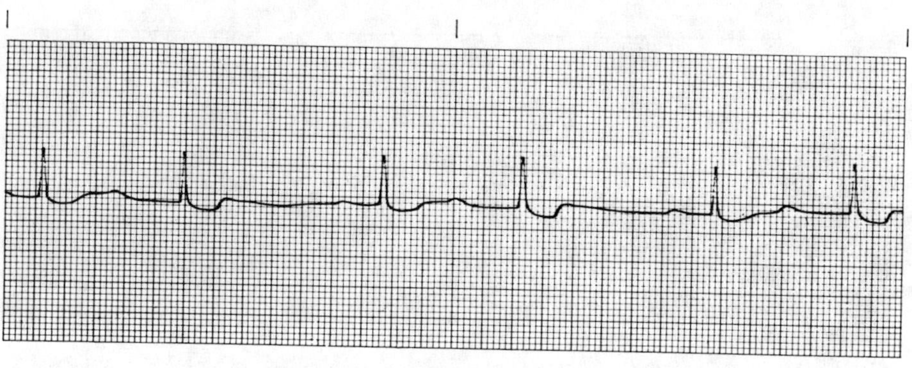

Figure 6–1. Rhythm Strip (Lead II)

Situation (refer to questions 6.83–6.87)

Your patient is male and is a 44-year-old loan officer at a local bank. His secretary called you because he has been feeling ill since he returned from lunch two hours ago. He describes his complaint as "indigestion," and you observe that he is also pale and diaphoretic. His blood pressure is 160/100, and his respirations are 28. You start him on oxygen by mask while you hook up the EKG. His rhythm is shown in Figure 6–2.

6.83 What is the *underlying* rhythm:
- **(a)** idioventricular rhythm
- **(b)** AV dissociation
- **(c)** normal sinus rhythm
- **(d)** pacemaker rhythm
- **(e)** atrial fibrillation

6.84 The ectopics are
- **(a)** unifocal PJCs
- **(b)** multifocal PVCs
- **(c)** bigeminy of PVCs
- **(d)** unifocal PVCs
- **(e)** bigeminy of PACs

6.85 Another abnormal feature of this strip is
- **(a)** prolonged PRI
- **(b)** elevated (ST) segments
- **(c)** absence of (Q) waves
- **(d)** pronounced (U) waves
- **(e)** absence of (R) waves

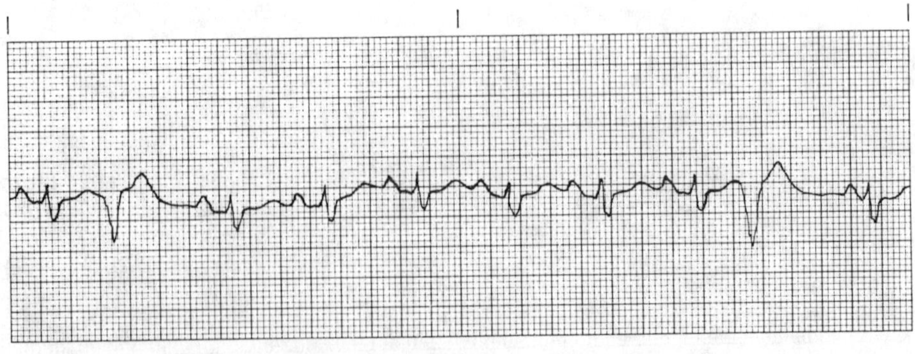

Figure 6–2. Rhythm Strip (Lead II)

6.86 Although the feature identified in 6.85 can be a sign of pathology, it might also be caused by
(a) 60-cycle interference
(b) "dead spots" in communication
(c) loose electrodes
(d) patient coughing
(e) intrinsic effect of telemetry

6.87 In addition to an IV and morphine for pain, this patient should also receive
(a) IV Lidocaine
(b) IV atropine
(c) IC sodium bicarbonate
(d) IC epinephrine
(e) IM calcium chloride

Situation (refer to questions 6.88–6.92)

Your patient is a 56-year-old male who is experiencing an oppressive pressure across his chest. He is dyspneic, pale, and nauseated. His wife tells you that he had a heart attack four years ago and had his gall bladder removed last year; other than that, he is in good health. His blood pressure is 98/60, pulse 80, and respirations 24. His EKG shows the rhythm of Figure 6–3.

6.88 This arrhythmia is
(a) ventricular tachycardia
(b) sinus rhythm with bigeminy of PVCs
(c) complete heart block
(d) Wenchebach (Mobitz I)
(e) idioventricular rhythm

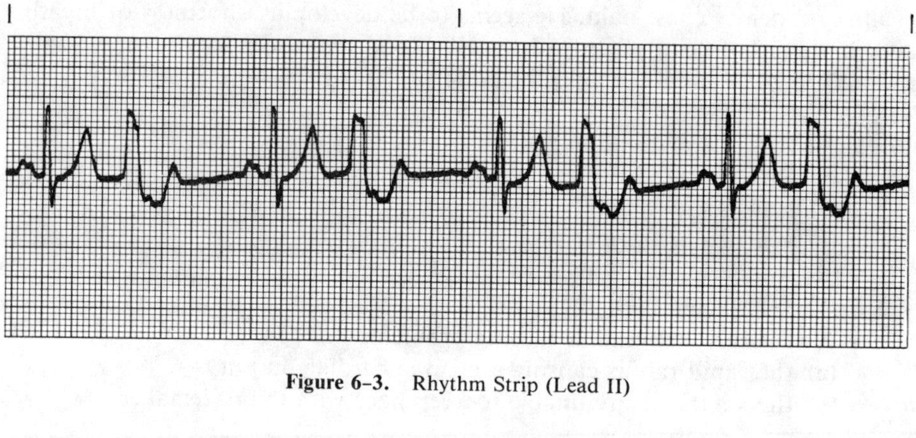

Figure 6–3. Rhythm Strip (Lead II)

6.89 How do you explain the disparity between the patient's pulse of 40 beats per minute and the rate shown on the EKG strip:
(a) the rate must have increased since the pulse was taken
(b) the rate increases and decreases with respirations
(c) you must have made an error when you counted the pulse initially
(d) the rate meter on the scope must be inaccurate
(e) the ectopics must not be producing pulse waves

6.90 Why is this arrhythmia so ominous:
(a) it is a sign of sinus node failure
(b) it can lead to severe heart blocks
(c) the rate can continue to drop
(d) it means the ventricles are extremely irritable
(e) it signals the onset of cardiogenic shock

6.91 What drug would you expect to use to treat this arrhythmia:
(a) atropine
(b) Isuprel
(c) Lidocaine
(d) epinephrine
(e) Valium

6.92 It is possible that the treatment in 6.91 would result in severe bradycardia. If this occurred, you would expect to
(a) give atropine
(b) give Isuprel
(c) prepare the patient for a pacemaker
(d) defibrillate
(e) do nothing; this is expected and will subside with time

Situation (refer to questions 6.93–6.97)

Your patient is a 42-year-old male who was awakened suddenly during the night with a feeling of "palpitations" in his chest. He has been in good health and denies chest pain. He seems to be developing shortness of breath and complains of being slightly dizzy. His blood pressure is 106/72, and respirations are 24. His EKG shows the pattern of Figure 6–4.

6.93 What is this arrhythmia:
(a) PACs
(b) sinus arrhythmia
(c) ventricular fibrillation
(d) wandering atrial pacemaker
(e) supraventricular tachycardia

6.94 Why is this arrhythmia causing problems:
(a) the rapid rate is causing a drop in cardiac output
(b) the ventricles are unable to keep pace with the pacemaker site

(c) the atria and the ventricles are dissociated
(d) the ventricles are so irritable that they are unreliable
(e) the atrial impulses aren't being conducted to the ventricles

6.95 Why would you want to treat this patient (instead of allowing the situation to a take care of itself):
(a) because this patient is probably having a concurrent MI
(b) because of the signs of dropping cardiac output
(c) because the patient is over 40
(d) because this arrhythmia is associated with a very high mortality rate
(e) because all arrhythmias should be treated as a precautionary measure

6.96 Which of the following would you consider for treating this arrhythmia:
(a) Lidocaine and possibly defibrillation
(b) oxygen, Lidocaine, and cardioversion
(c) vagotonic maneuvers and possibly Digoxin
(d) Inderal, defibrillation, and possibly Lidocaine
(e) dopamine, Aramine, or Levophed

6.97 On the way to the hospital, your patient appears much better. What would you watch for as an early sign that the problem might be starting again:
(a) supraventricular ectopics
(b) first-degree heart block
(c) PVCs
(d) sinus arrest
(e) sinus block

Situation (refer to questions 6.98–6.102)

You respond to the beach, where lifeguards are performing CPR on a teenage male. Your assessment reveals strong carotid pulses with CPR, but no

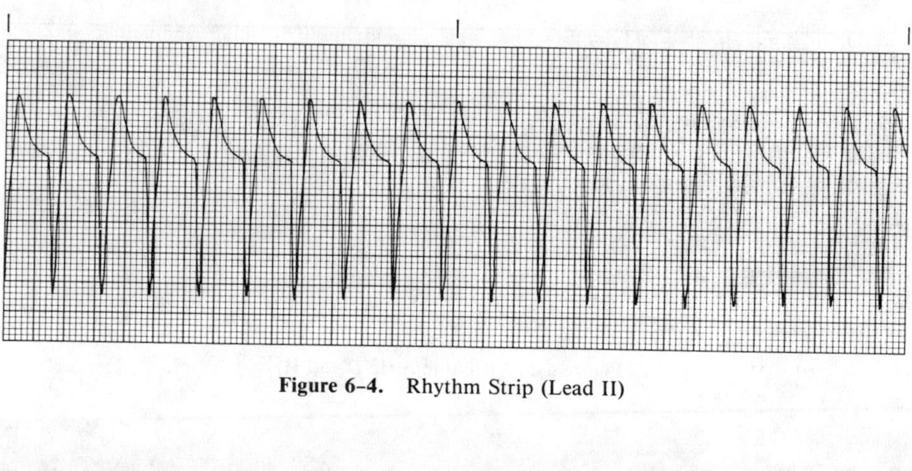

Figure 6-4. Rhythm Strip (Lead II)

pulses when CPR is withheld. The patient has no B/P and no spontaneous respirations. His EKG pattern is shown in Figure 6–5.

6.98 What is this arrhythmia:
(a) ventricular fibrillation
(b) electromechanical dissociation
(c) coarse atrial fib/flutter
(d) idioventricular rhythm
(e) massage artifact

6.99 Of the following, which would you do *last:*
(a) establish a good airway
(b) ventilate with positive pressure
(c) give Lidocaine
(d) give epinephrine
(e) defibrillate

6.100 Which of the following would *not* be included in your treatment of this patient:
(a) immobilize the spine
(b) insert an N/G tube
(c) evacuate water from the lungs
(d) keep patient warm
(e) suction the airway

6.101 You defibrillate the patient and the rhythm converts to idioventricular rhythm with a rate of 28. Which of the following is *most* appropriate:
(a) atropine, Isuprel, or epinephrine
(b) Isuprel and repeated defibrillation
(c) epinephrine, calcium chloride, and Digoxin
(d) Lidocaine followed by Isuprel if necessary
(e) transport immediately for a pacemaker

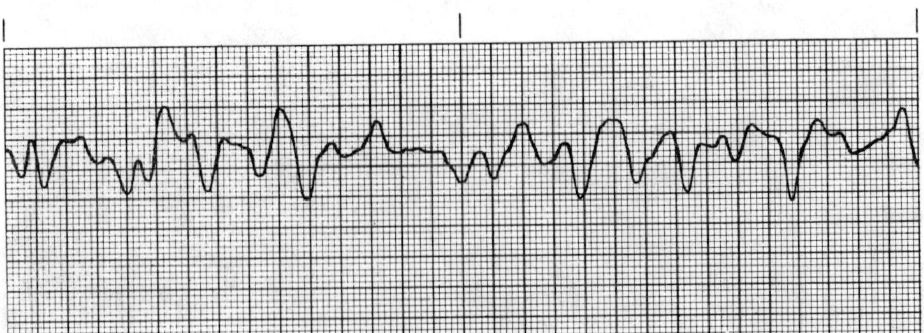

Figure 6–5. Rhythm Strip (Lead II)

6.102 You eventually resuscitate the patient to a point where he has good peripheral pulses and spontaneous respirations. Which of the following would you *not* do:

(a) continue giving high flow oxygen
(b) monitor closely for EKG changes
(c) repeat the sodium bicarbonate at 10-minute intervals
(d) collect a sample of the water and take it with you to the hospital
(e) examine the patient for associated illness/injury

Situation (refer to questions 6.103–6.107)

Your patient is a 68-year-old female who was involved in a minor car accident. Other than a broken ankle, she has no apparent injuries. Her vital signs are B/P 138/90, pulse 120, respirations 24. Her skin is warm and dry, although she is slightly shaken up. Her EKG shows the pattern of Figure 6–6.

6.103 What is this arrhythmia:

(a) atrial fibrillation
(b) atrial flutter
(c) ventricular fibrillation
(d) ventricular tachycardia
(e) sinus tachycardia with PACs

6.104 Which of the following statements about this arrhythmia is most correct:

(a) it is a relatively benign pattern that is fairly common, especially in elderly people
(b) it is life-threatening when the rate exceeds 100 beats per minute
(c) it is caused by damage to the ventricular conduction system
(d) it is often associated with an MI
(e) the fluctuation in rate is associated with respirations

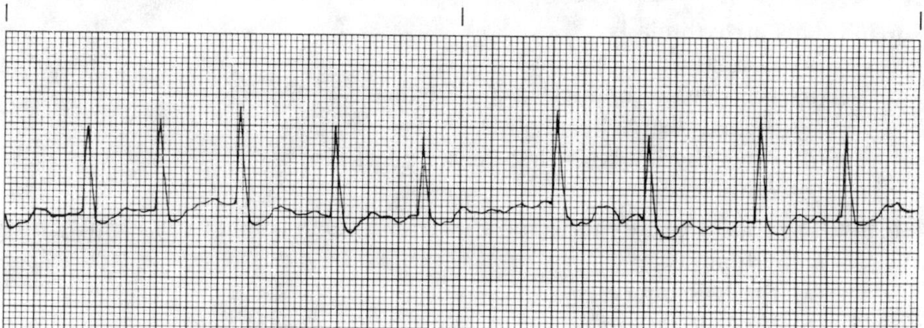

Figure 6–6. Rhythm Strip (Lead II)

6.105 Which of the following is the most likely complication of this arrhythmia:
(a) heart block
(b) ventricular irritability
(c) pulmonary embolus
(d) bundle branch block
(e) primary asystole

6.106 Your field treatment of this patient would include an IV of LR TKO, oxygen, splinting the ankle, and
(a) morphine sulfate to ease respiratory effort and help alleviate pain
(b) Lidocaine to reduce ventricular irritability
(c) cardioversion to stimulate a more reliable pacemaker
(d) defibrillation to override the irritable focus
(e) none of the above; no further treatment is indicated

6.107 After loading the patient into the ambulance, you reassess her vital signs. Although her blood pressure remains the same, her pulse has slowed to 110 and her respirations are down to 18. You conclude that
(a) she needs more oxygen
(b) this is an expected result of the drugs that you have given her
(c) it is not unusual for the rate to fluctuate this widely in this arrhythmia
(d) she is probably calming down after the accident
(e) she has taken a turn for the worse and the hospital should be notified

Situation (refer to questions 6.108–6.112)

Your patient is a 73-year-old male with no history of serious medical illness. His wife called you because he has had repeated episodes of dizziness and fainting within the last few hours. When you monitor the EKG, you find the pattern of Figure 6–7.

6.108 This arrhythmia is
(a) normal sinus rhythm
(b) ventricular conduction disturbance
(c) second-degree heart block
(d) sinus rhythm with first-degree heart block
(e) sinus block

6.109 The EKG feature that is most instrumental in helping you identify this arrhythmia is
(a) the R-R interval
(b) the P-R interval
(c) the P-P interval

(d) the Q-T interval
(e) the S-T segment

6.110 Your main concern in this patient is the possibility that he will develop
(a) secondary pump failure
(b) electromechanical dissociation
(c) ventricular fibrillation
(d) atrial irritability
(e) further heart block

6.111 The distinction between this arrhythmia and a complete heart block is that CHB
(a) involves AV dissociation
(b) causes fewer complications
(c) has a constant P-R interval
(d) has an irregular R-R interval
(e) has elevated S-T segments

6.112 The most appropriate treatment for this arrhythmia is
(a) IV, atropine, and immediate transport
(b) oxygen, IV, and Lidocaine
(c) oxygen, IV, and close monitoring
(d) atropine, Isuprel, and possibly epinephrine
(e) sodium bicarbonate and calcium chloride

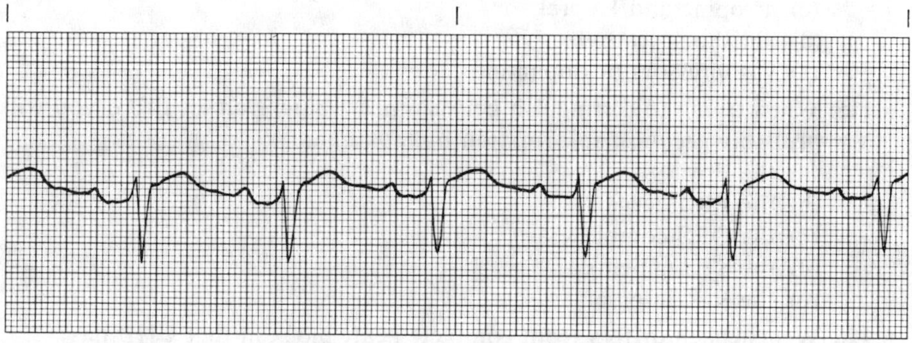

Figure 6–7. Rhythm Strip (Lead II)

Situation (refer to questions 6.113–6.117)

You have stabilized a male who has been having Stokes-Adams attacks. He is in sinus rhythm with first-degree heart block, but en route to the hospital his rhythm changes, as shown in Figure 6–8.

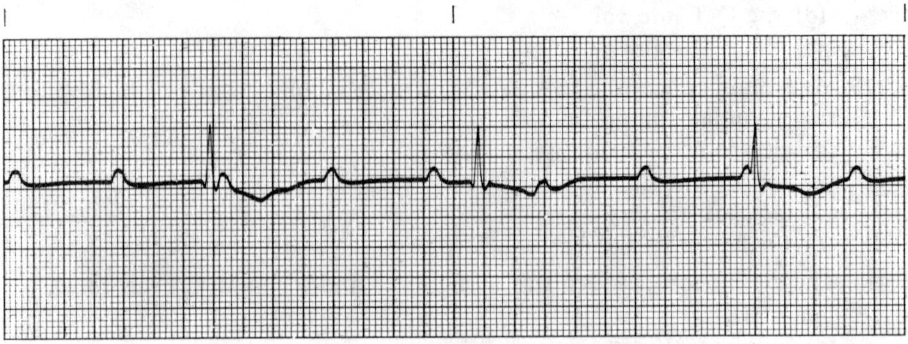

Figure 6–8. Rhythm Strip (Lead II)

6.113 What is this arrhythmia:
- **(a)** sinus rhythm with first-degree heart block
- **(b)** classic second-degree (Mobitz II)
- **(c)** Wenchebach (Mobitz I)
- **(d)** third-degree heart block (CHB)
- **(e)** electromechanical dissociation

6.114 The patient begins to lose consciousness and his blood pressure drops. You should consider
- **(a)** defibrillation
- **(b)** Lidocaine
- **(c)** atropine and Isuprel
- **(d)** antishock trousers
- **(e)** vasopressors or dopamine

6.115 When trying to distinguish between heart blocks on an EKG, you will probably get *most* information by looking at
- **(a)** the P waves
- **(b)** the PR intervals
- **(c)** the QRS complexes
- **(d)** the ST segments
- **(e)** the R-R intervals

6.116 Wenchebach differs from complete heart block in that CHB has
- **(a)** regular R-R intervals
- **(b)** a constant PRI
- **(c)** a faster rate
- **(d)** a normal QRS duration
- **(e)** upright P waves

6.117 Classic second-degree heart block differs from both Wenchebach and third-degree heart block in that classic second-degree heart block has
- **(a)** more P waves that QRS complexes
- **(b)** a slower-than-normal ventricular rate

(c) a normal QRS duration
(d) irregular P-P intervals
(e) constant PR intervals

Situation (refer to questions 6.118–6.122)

A female is employed by a commercial greenhouse and has been working all morning in a hothouse, feeding and disinfecting the plants. She was fine when seen about an hour ago but is now incoherent, drooling, and experiencing mild skeletal muscle tremors and has been incontinent of urine. Her blood pressure is 124/88, and respirations are 20. Her EKG is shown in Figure 6–9.

6.118 What is this EKG pattern:
- **(a)** normal sinus rhythm
- **(b)** sinus bradycardia
- **(c)** junctional rhythm
- **(d)** second-degree heart block
- **(e)** idioventricular rhythm

6.119 Which of the following is *most* likely the cause of this patient's difficulty:
- **(a)** this arrhythmia is not capable of maintaining adequate perfusion
- **(b)** the patient has experienced a seizure and is now in a postictal state
- **(c)** the symptoms suggest neurological trauma; you should look for supporting evidence
- **(d)** the patient is probably suffering from organophosphate poisoning
- **(e)** you have inadequate information to formulate a diagnosis at this time

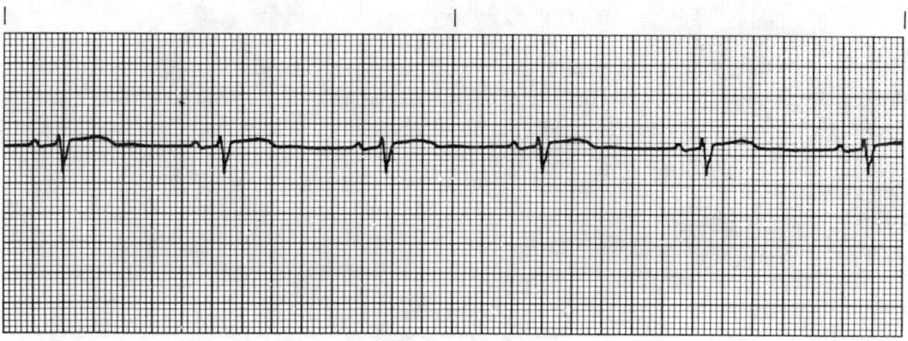

Figure 6–9. Rhythm Strip (Lead II)

6.120 How would you treat this patient:
- **(a)** send a 12-lead EKG to the hospital
- **(b)** give Valium to control the muscle tremors
- **(c)** give atropine to reverse the parasympathetic effects
- **(d)** start an IV and insert an EOA
- **(e)** transport for pacemaker implantation

6.121 Following your treatment, the patient improves dramatically. You should
- **(a)** watch for ectopics
- **(b)** watch for a drop in blood pressure
- **(c)** administer sodium bicarbonate
- **(d)** watch for a recurrence of initial symptoms
- **(e)** apply a cervical collar to stabilize the spine

6.122 It is imperative that this patient be transported to the hospital because she
- **(a)** requires an additional drug to treat this problem
- **(b)** needs further diagnostic studies
- **(c)** needs surgery
- **(d)** should be hospitalized for observation
- **(e)** will require rehabilitative therapy

Situation (refer to questions 6.123–6.127)

Your patient is a young male with a suspected heroin overdose. He is unconscious, with blood pressure of 70/58 and shallow respirations at a rate of 6 per minute. His EKG shows the pattern of Figure 6–10.

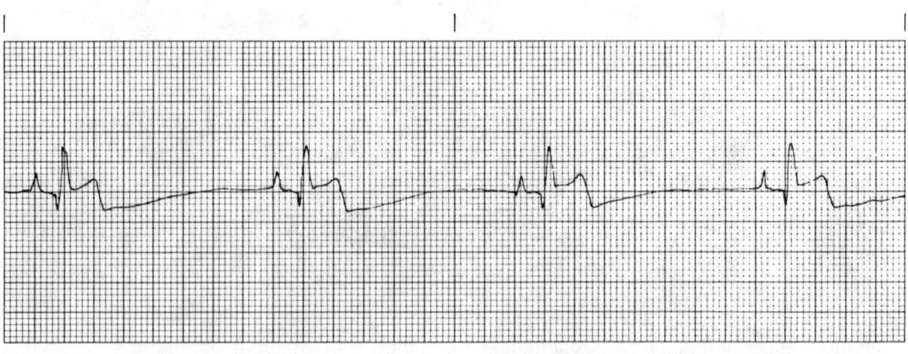

Figure 6–10. Rhythm Strip (Lead II)

6.123 This arrhythmia is most likely
- **(a)** sinus bradycardia
- **(b)** fine atrial fibrillation
- **(c)** junctional escape rhythm
- **(d)** idioventricular rhythm
- **(e)** AV dissociation

6.124 The drug of choice for this patient is
- **(a)** atropine
- **(b)** Isuprel
- **(c)** epinephrine
- **(d)** Narcan
- **(e)** calcium chloride

6.125 You should expect to see a response to this drug within
- **(a)** 2 minutes
- **(b)** 2 to 10 minutes
- **(c)** 30 minutes to 1 hour
- **(d)** 4 hours
- **(e)** 24 hours

6.126 If the arrhythmia persists after the patient responds to the initial drug therapy, you would consider giving
- **(a)** atropine
- **(b)** Valium
- **(c)** Digoxin
- **(d)** Lidocaine
- **(e)** Inderal

6.127 En route to the hospital, you might expect the patient to experience
- **(a)** complete heart block
- **(b)** recurrence of the initial syndrome
- **(c)** hypertension
- **(d)** laryngospasm
- **(e)** seizure activity

Situation (refer to questions 6.128–6.132)

You respond to the scene of a minor traffic accident. Your only patient is a 62-year-old female who has bumped her head. She is very shaken and is complaining of "dizziness and tingling." Her blood pressure is 112/64, pulse is 80, and respirations are 32 and shallow. Her head wound appears minor, so you connect her to the cardiac monitor and find the arrhythmia shown in Figure 6–11.

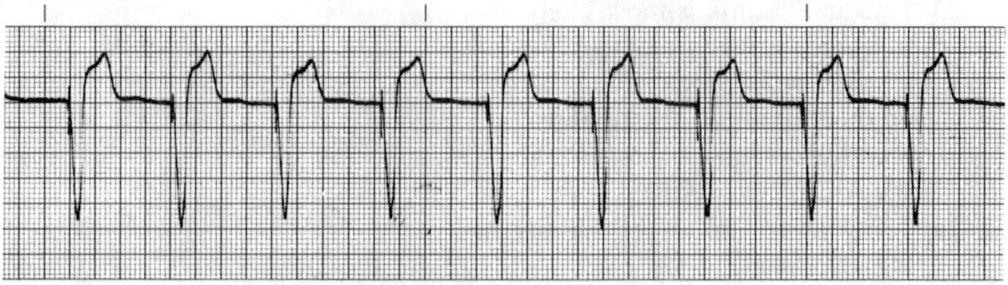

Figure 6–11. Rhythm Strip (Lead II)

6.128 This arrhythmia is
- **(a)** idioventricular rhythm
- **(b)** complete heart block
- **(c)** atrial fibrillation with bundle branch block
- **(d)** junctional escape rhythm
- **(e)** ventricular pacemaker

6.129 In order to confirm your interpretation of this arrhythmia, you might consider
- **(a)** cardioversion and defibrillation
- **(b)** carotid sinus massage to see if the rate changes
- **(c)** changing leads to visualize blips
- **(d)** atropine to stimulate a higher pacemaker
- **(e)** Lidocaine to eliminate the ventricular focus

6.130 Since you know that this arrhythmia does not normally produce symptoms, you look for other causes for the patient's complaints. She has no abnormality on the neurological assessment. Your next most likely suspicion is that she is suffering from
- **(a)** TIA
- **(b)** hypoxia
- **(c)** seizure disorder
- **(d)** hyperventilation
- **(e)** hypoglycemia

6.131 Following discussion with your hospital, you proceed to treat the patient by
- **(a)** having her breathe into a paper bag
- **(b)** giving high flow oxygen
- **(c)** ventilating with positive pressure oxygen
- **(d)** starting an IV and giving dextrose
- **(e)** giving oral carbohydrate solution

6.132 En route to the hospital, you should do all of the following *except*
(a) monitor the EKG rhythm
(b) monitor respiration closely
(c) insert an oropharyngeal airway
(d) reassess vital signs
(e) auscultate lungs

Situation (refer to questions 6.133–6.137)

You respond to a private home to find a young male unconscious on the living room floor. There are indications of a party in the room, but no one else is there. You note that the patient's respirations are very shallow and slow, so you initiate positive pressure ventilation until a firefighter takes over for you. The patient has a weak pulse with a rate of about 80 and blood pressure of 114/72. The monitor shows the rhythm in Figure 6–12.

6.133 What is this arrhythmia:
(a) AV dissociation
(b) accelerated junctional rhythm
(c) wandering atrial pacemaker
(d) electromechanical dissociation
(e) Wenchebach

6.134 As you are examining the patient for injuries, you find melting ice cubes inside his jeans and discolorations along the veins of his forearm. You suspect that he is suffering from drug overdose and anticipate administering
(a) Ipecac
(b) 50 percent dextrose
(c) Levophed
(d) Physostigmine
(e) Narcan

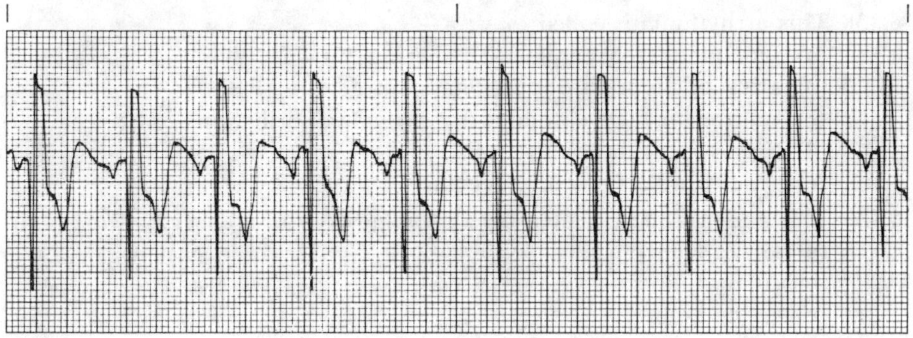

Figure 6–12. Rhythm Strip (Lead II)

6.135 Since you know that this drug is expected to elicit a very rapid response, you will withhold
- **(a)** starting the IV
- **(b)** transmitting the EKG to the hospital
- **(c)** inserting an esophageal obturator airway
- **(d)** resuscitative measures
- **(e)** preparations for transport

6.136 Within minutes of administration your patient is aroused and becoming abrasive. His respirations have improved, and other vital signs are stable. How would you expect his EKG rhythm to respond:
- **(a)** improve and return to normal
- **(b)** improve somewhat but be permanently damaged
- **(c)** stabilize in this pattern but not return to normal
- **(d)** deteriorate unless antiarrhythmic agents are administered
- **(e)** remain unstable and continue to change unpredictably

6.137 Just after loading your patient into the ambulance, you note that he is having occasional PACs. His vital signs remain stable, and his level of consciousness has not changed. Which of the following might you consider to reduce the PACs:
- **(a)** Lidocaine
- **(b)** atropine
- **(c)** repeated Narcan
- **(d)** high-flow oxygen
- **(e)** no treatment; PACs don't require it

Situation (refer to questions 6.138–6.142)

Your patient, a male, is a 57-year-old gas station attendant who collapsed during a robbery attempt. He is in cardiac arrest. Your initial assessment of EKG activity shows the pattern in Figure 6–13.

6.138 This arrhythmia is called
- **(a)** junctional tachycardia with aberrancy
- **(b)** a run of premature junctional contractions (PJCs)
- **(c)** ventricular tachycardia into ventricular fibrillation
- **(d)** supraventricular tachycardia
- **(e)** atrial fibrillation with aberrancy

6.139 This patient is best treated by continuing your resuscitation efforts and
- **(a)** giving epinephrine
- **(b)** giving Lidocaine
- **(c)** giving Isuprel
- **(d)** giving calcium chloride
- **(e)** defibrillating

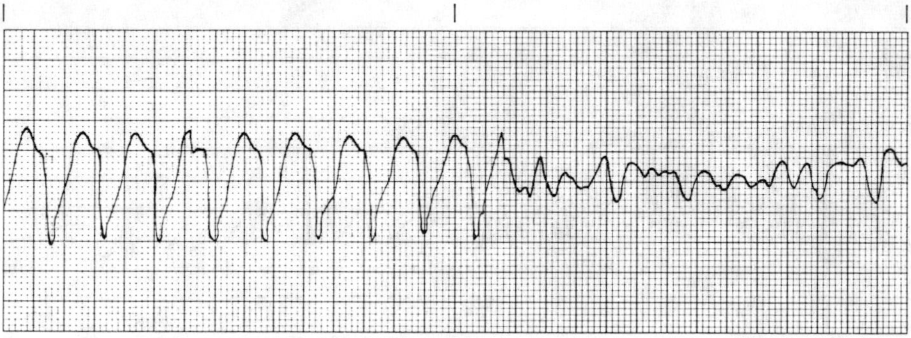

Figure 6–13. Rhythm Strip (Lead II)

6.140 What one clinical factor might have altered your choice of treatment for this patient:
(a) age
(b) level of consciousness
(c) presence of trauma
(d) physical surroundings
(e) medical history

6.141 Following conversion, your patient reverts to a sinus rhythm with a rate of 68. Considering the original arrhythmia, you would expect to get an order for
(a) Isuprel
(b) sodium bicarbonate
(c) Inderal
(d) Lidocaine
(e) Aminophylline

6.142 Although your patient's perfusion has improved, you might also expect to get an order for something to augment cardiovascular status. The most likely choice for general cardiovascular support would be
(a) dopamine
(b) Inderal
(c) volume IV fluids
(d) rotating tourniquets
(e) epinephrine

Situation (refer to questions 6.143–6.147)

You are spending some time in the CCU as part of your continuing education program. One of the patients is a 66-year-old female. She has used digitalis for several years to control mild congestive heart failure but has recently been admitted for a work-up. Her monitor shows the pattern in Figure 6–14.

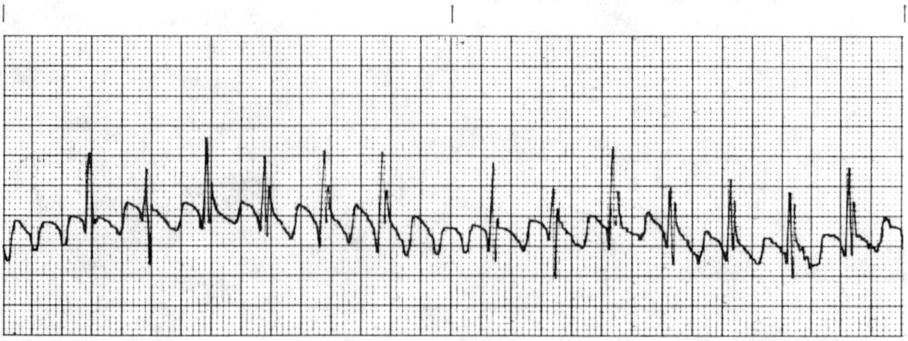

Figure 6–14. Rhythm Strip (Lead II)

6.143 This arrhythmia is
- **(a)** atrial fibrillation
- **(b)** atrial flutter
- **(c)** ventricular fibrillation
- **(d)** complete heart block
- **(e)** Wenchebach

6.144 Although the QRS has a normal measurement, it has an unusual configuration. This is probably caused by
- **(a)** bundle branch block
- **(b)** aberrant conduction through the ventricles
- **(c)** F waves superimposed on the QRS complex
- **(d)** an AV conduction defect
- **(e)** AV dissociation

6.145 The irregularity of the R-R interval is caused by
- **(a)** variable conduction through the AV node
- **(b)** an unreliable ventricular focus
- **(c)** an irregular sinus pacemaker
- **(d)** parasympathetic influence with respirations
- **(e)** patient movement

6.146 If this arrhythmia began causing symptoms, you would consider treating it with
- **(a)** defibrillation
- **(b)** cardioversion
- **(c)** Lidocaine
- **(d)** atropine
- **(e)** a pacemaker

6.147 Your proposed treatment might present a problem because
- **(a)** the patient is 66 years old
- **(b)** she has respiratory difficulty

(c) she has been taking digitalis
(d) this arrhythmia is exceedingly difficult to convert
(e) this treatment usually has severe complications

Situation (refer to questions 6.148–6.152)

You and your partner are giving a public relations demonstration at the local parent-teacher meeting. A male teacher volunteers to be your "patient." When you hook him up to the EKG, you find that he has the arrhythmia shown in Figure 6–15.

6.148 What is this arrhythmia:
(a) wandering atrial pacemaker
(b) premature atrial contractions
(c) premature ventricular contractions
(d) atrial fibrillation
(e) sinus arrhythmia

6.149 In this arrhythmia, the changing R-R intervals correlate with changes in the patient's
(a) movement
(b) emotional state
(c) breathing
(d) level of consciousness
(e) blood pressure

6.150 This arrhythmia differs from atrial fibrillation in that atrial fibrillation does not have
(a) rate changes
(b) P waves
(c) T waves

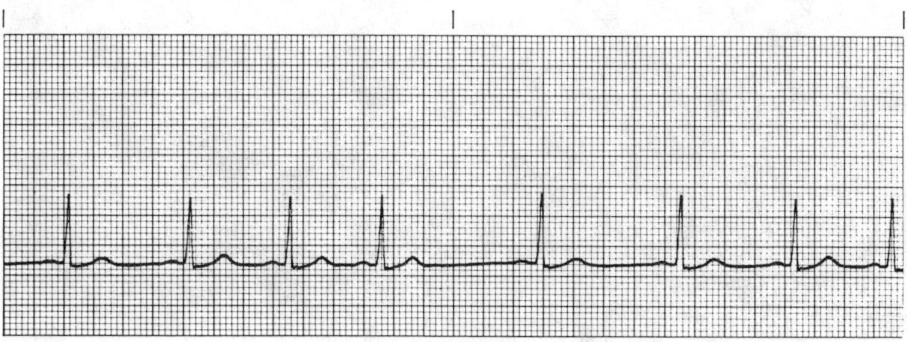

Figure 6–15. Rhythm Strip (Lead II)

(d) QRS complexes
(e) ST segments

6.151 Which of the following statements about this arrhythmia is *not* true:
(a) it requires long-term monitoring by the family physician
(b) it is common in children
(c) it is found in about one-third of the general population
(d) it does not produce clinical symptoms
(e) it requires no treatment

6.152 Your treatment for this patient will include
(a) IV, oxygen, and transport
(b) Lidocaine
(c) referral to private physician
(d) only oxygen
(e) no treatment is required

Situation (refer to questions 6.153–6.157)

You are in the middle of a cardiac arrest situation. You have given epinephrine and sodium bicarbonate and have defibrillated three times. Following the last defibrillation, the patient, a male, converted to the arrhythmia of Figure 6–16.

6.153 This arrhythmia shows a rapid ventricular focus going into
(a) complete heart block
(b) asystole
(c) ventricular standstill
(d) sinus arrest
(e) ventricular escape rhythm

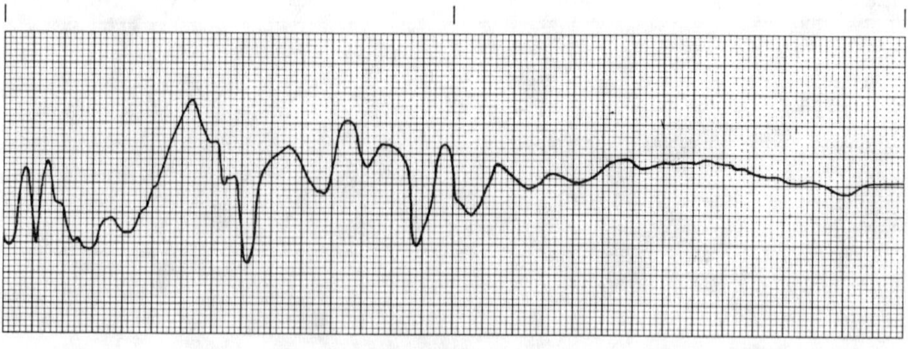

Figure 6–16. Rhythm Strip (Lead II)

6.154 While the patient is in this rhythm, he is most likely to be
(a) conscious and asymptomatic
(b) conscious but extremely apprehensive
(c) slowly regaining consciousness
(d) unconscious but perfusing well
(e) pulseless and apneic

6.155 Your objective in treating this arrhythmia would be to
(a) suppress ventricular ectopics
(b) increase the rate of the SA mode
(c) stimulate a junctional or ventricular pacemaker
(d) improve conduction through the AV node
(e) either (c) or (d)

6.156 In order to improve this arrhythmia, you would consider giving
(a) epinephrine
(b) Lidocaine
(c) calcium chloride
(d) Inderal
(e) Digoxin

6.157 Of the following, which would be *least* likely to be included in the management of this patient:
(a) Aminophylline
(b) dopamine
(c) antishock trousers
(d) nasogastric tube
(e) suctioning

ANSWER KEY

6.1 d	**6.16** a	**6.31** d	**6.46** c
6.2 c	**6.17** b	**6.32** c	**6.47** e
6.3 d	**6.18** c	**6.33** e	**6.48** d
6.4 b	**6.19** b	**6.34** a	**6.49** e
6.5 d	**6.20** c	**6.35** a	**6.50** d
6.6 c	**6.21** e	**6.36** b	**6.51** d
6.7 a	**6.22** d	**6.37** d	**6.52** b
6.8 d	**6.23** a	**6.38** c	**6.53** d
6.9 b	**6.24** b	**6.39** b	**6.54** a
6.10 b	**6.25** b	**6.40** a	**6.55** d
6.11 c	**6.26** b	**6.41** b	**6.56** c
6.12 e	**6.27** c	**6.42** c	**6.57** b
6.13 c	**6.28** c	**6.43** b	**6.58** d
6.14 a	**6.29** d	**6.44** e	**6.59** d
6.15 d	**6.30** d	**6.45** c	**6.60** e

6.61 a
6.62 c
6.63 d
6.64 a
6.65 c
6.66 a
6.67 c
6.68 c
6.69 e
6.70 b
6.71 e
6.72 b
6.73 a
6.74 a
6.75 c
6.76 a
6.77 e
6.78 c
6.79 d
6.80 b
6.81 d
6.82 d
6.83 c
6.84 d
6.85 b
6.86 e
6.87 a
6.88 b
6.89 e
6.90 d
6.91 c
6.92 a
6.93 e
6.94 a
6.95 b
6.96 c
6.97 a
6.98 a
6.99 c
6.100 c
6.101 a
6.102 c
6.103 a
6.104 a
6.105 c
6.106 e
6.107 d
6.108 d
6.109 b
6.110 e
6.111 a
6.112 c
6.113 d
6.114 c
6.115 b
6.116 a
6.117 e
6.118 b
6.119 d
6.120 c
6.121 d
6.122 a
6.123 c
6.124 d
6.125 a
6.126 a
6.127 b
6.128 e
6.129 c
6.130 d
6.131 a
6.132 c
6.133 b
6.134 e
6.135 c
6.136 a
6.137 d
6.138 c
6.139 e
6.140 b
6.141 d
6.142 a
6.143 b
6.144 c
6.145 a
6.146 b
6.147 c
6.148 e
6.149 c
6.150 b
6.151 a
6.152 e
6.153 b
6.154 e
6.155 e
6.156 a
6.157 a

7

CENTRAL NERVOUS SYSTEM EMERGENCIES

CASE STUDY 7A: MR. B. BAKER

Your paramedic unit responds to a hang glider accident on a weekend afternoon. When you arrive, there is a crowd around the patient, a male, who is lying on the ground. As you approach, you can see someone performing mouth-to-mouth resuscitation on the victim. The calm rescuer states that there is a strong pulse but that the patient is not breathing. Your partner quickly confirms that the patient is in fact apneic, but a pulse is present. A witness tells you that the hapless pilot lost control of his hang glider at about 50 feet and struck the ground head first. When they reached him, he was unconscious and not breathing.

On the basis of this information how would you now control the airway:

1. hyperextend the neck by using head-tilt method
2. attempt to intubate the trachea through the mouth
3. use a jaw-thrust or chin-lift method
4. place a pillow under the shoulders

A patient who is apneic following trauma immediately suggests either airway obstruction or damage to the cervical spinal cord above C–4. Severe injury or transection of the cord above this level prevents stimulation of the diaphragm by the phrenic nerve, resulting in respiratory paralysis. The airway should be controlled by a procedure, such as jaw-thrust or chin-lift, which does not cause unnecessary manipulation of the cervical spine.

After the airway is opened, your partner inserts an oral airway and hyperventilates the patient with a bag/mask device to which high flow oxygen has been connected. You place EKG monitor electrodes on his chest and observe a normal sinus rhythm. The blood pressure is 132/90. The pupils are midpoint, equal, and reactive. There are swelling and deformity in the right upper arm, suggesting a fracture. The abdomen is soft, and breath sounds are bilaterally clear in all fields. Within a short period, your previously unconscious patient wakens. He is slightly confused and does not recall his accident. His extremities remain flaccid, and he is unable to move his limbs voluntarily. There also are complete loss of sensation below his shoulders and no unilateral findings.

This physical exam suggests

1. basilar skull fracture
2. severe spinal cord injury
3. subdural hematoma
4. hyperventilation syndrome

These physical findings point to a severe injury to the spinal cord. Loss of consciousness may have resulted from a head injury sustained in the fall. While return of consciousness may have been a natural progression from such a blow, it possibly resulted from hyperventilation carried out by the paramedics, which decreased cerebral hypoxia.

In the face of such grim neurological findings, you and your partner realize that careful movement and immobilization of this patient are crucial. A cervical collar is applied first. Next, a splint is applied to the right arm to stabilize that injury. A scoop stretcher is then placed underneath the patient and sandbags placed along each side of his head. Finally, wide cloth tape is applied across his forehead and anchored on either side of the stretcher. Your partner continues to ventilate with the bag/mask, because there is no spontaneous respiratory effort. A recheck of the patient's pulse and blood pressure shows them to be within normal limits. After carefully considering your patient's present condition, you decide to request transport by helicopter to the nearby regional trauma center.

Why is a helicopter indicated for this patient:

1. rapid transport to a specialized spinal cord center
2. smoothness of ride by air versus land ambulance
3. speed of transport to the across-town facility
4. all of the above

Although you may have to wait for the helicopter to arrive, this inconvenience is outweighed by all of these benefits.

Within 10 minutes the drone of the Aerospatiale "Alouette" helicopter can be heard. The crowd of bystanders is cordoned back, and the helicopter lands gently on the grass about 100 feet away. A physician and flight nurse climb out of the aircraft and join you and your partner. Your partner briefs the physician on the patient's status, and the physician appears favorably impressed with the immobilization of the patient's neck and spine. After performing an initial neurological exam, the physician directs the patient to be loaded aboard the helicopter.

Discussion

Spinal injuries can range anywhere from cervical muscle spasm (i.e., whiplash) to lesion of the spinal cord itself. Often, in the absence of any obvious neurologic trauma, cautious handling and proper splinting may prevent further injury. Stories of well-meaning individuals (including paramedical personnel) who may have been responsible for inflicting post-trauma injury are always disturbing. Priorities in handling patients with suspected spinal injuries include airway management, cardiovascular stabilization if necessary, proper spinal immobilization, a check for associated injuries, and smooth, low-speed transport. A neurological field exam is always appropriate in establishing a baseline for in-hospital observations. It should include respiratory status, level of consciousness, pupils, movement of all extremities, and sensation to touch. All such observations should be carefully recorded for later reference.

In following up on your patient, you find that he did, in fact, have a fractured cervical spine with accompanying spinal cord damage. His neck is surgically stabilized, but he remains on a respirator at this point, three weeks after his injury.

CASE STUDY 7B: MS. J. ELLIS

Your paramedic unit is dispatched to a female having convulsions. It is only a brief two-minute response from your station to the small mobile home park. Once inside the park, however, you are annoyed by the many speed bumps across the streets, designed to prevent excessive speeding. Not only does it slow your response time as you creep slowly over the bumps, but it will create a very uncomfortable ride for the patient when you ride to the hospital. The mobile home is located, and you shut off the red lights as you stop. Once inside the trailer, you and your partner find the patient, a female in her early 30s, still actively seizing on the living room floor. As you set down your equipment, you note that her arms and legs are bilaterally outstretched and trembling somewhat. Her jaw is clenched, and saliva is drooling down her cheek. You would probably describe her seizure as

1. tonic
2. clonic
3. petit mal
4. Jacksonian

The paramedic team should be able to describe the type of seizure. Obviously this is grand mal, which refers to the fact that it is a generalized body seizure. However, it may further be described by the activity of major muscle groups and especially the extremities. Tonic refers to a state of muscle contraction in either flexion or extension and most closely describes your patient's seizure. Clonic describes a patient whose arms and legs are alternating between contraction and relaxation. A Jacksonian seizure progresses from one muscle group to another.

As you quickly begin to examine your patient, her seizure subsides; you start her on high flow oxygen. However, she remains unconscious and unresponsive to verbal stimulus. A firm pinch of her trapezius muscle also elicits no response. Her pupils are midpoint and react equally to light. Her respiratory rate is 24 and unlabored. Pulse is 120 and strong. Blood pressure is 136/82. Her skin is warm and moist, her color is normal. You suction a slight amount of excess saliva from her mouth and insert an oropharyngeal airway. Just as you insert the airway, the patient begins to seize again. Meanwhile your partner has spoken to the woman's husband and discovered that she had a seizure two months ago. She has no other known illnesses, medications, or allergies. This present seizure is also tonic in nature. Your partner immediately requests an IV order to keep open. In addition you are told to give 10 mg Valium (diazepam) slow IV.

Which of the following side effects should be foremost in your mind while administering Valium:

1. cardiac arrhythmias
2. transient hypertension
3. respiratory depression
4. numbness and tingling in the extremities

Valium is a central nervous system depressant. Its major side effect is respiratory depression, since the respiratory center is located in the brain stem. It is generally used in the field for recurrent seizure activity (status epilepticus), precardioversion sedation, and acute stress reactions.

Your first attempt at the IV is not successful, but on a second try dark red blood flashes into the cannula, signifying that you are in the vein. You hastily tape the cannula and tubing down to prevent dislodgment. With an alcohol pad you swab the rubber injection site on the IV tubing and slowly start injecting the clear, yellow-tinged drug from the syringe. *(Note:* Generally, drugs should be administered only if they are clear and colorless. Diazepam is one of a few drugs that normally has slight color.)

Which of the following methods is most acceptable when giving IV Valium:

1. pinch IV tubing, inject total amount ordered, and run IV wide open
2. open IV to rapid drip and slowly titrate 2.5 mg increments over one minute
3. inject directly into any available dorsal hand vein
4. dilute with 100 ml 5 percent D/W in Volutrol

Large doses of Valium may be required to control grand mal seizures that are not self-limiting. However, it is always titrated slowly to prevent respiratory depression or arrest. Drugs that are given slow IV (not as a drip dilution) may be safely administered by (1) pinching the tubing, injecting a small increment, then flushing the tubing or (2) opening the IV line to a fast drip and slowly injecting the medication to the desired effect, watching for any backup of the IV solution in the drip chamber. While occasionally given direct IV, Valium is extremely painful for the patient, especially when injected into a small vein.

After 10 mg of Valium your patient stops seizing but remains unresponsive. Within four minutes she begins to seize again, and the hospital orders an additional 10 mg titrated to effect. The patient's seizure appears the same as the two that you have witnessed. There is no localized or unilateral activity. With 20 mg Valium on board, the seizure stops. Vital signs remain the same, although the respiratory rate increases following each seizure. The patient is placed on the gurney and taken to the waiting ambulance. She is responding purposefully to pain, since she shrugs her shoulder away when you pinch the trapezius. Oxygen is running at 6 1 by cannula, and the monitor shows a borderline sinus tachycardia.

As you review possible causes for her seizure, which of the following would you most likely dismiss:

1. epilepsy
2. toxemia
3. hypoglycemia
4. overdose

All of the choices, as well as many others, can precipitate a grand mal seizure. In the last trimester of pregnancy, toxemia can produce seizures; however, there is no indication of pregnancy.

At the hospital your patient begins to become more responsive and is conscious but disoriented. She remembers nothing about her seizures and wants to see her husband. You recognize this slightly decreased level of consciousness as postictal, normal for a patient who has had a grand mal seizure. Lab tests ordered by the ER physician are negative, and your patient is sent to radiology for a CAT (computerized axial tomography) scan.

Discussion

Few medical emergencies are as frightening for the unexperienced to observe as a grand mal seizure. Often the patient becomes a spectacle as onlookers watch the victim writhe. Unfortunately, the cause of a seizure is frequently impossible to determine. While the first attack may be the only one that a patient may ever experience, it may also herald a lifetime of potential seizure activity.

Treatment of a seizure patient in the field is directed primarily at managing the airway and protecting the patient from self-inflicted trauma. A "bite-stick" can be beneficial if it can be placed between the teeth to protect the tongue and maintain the airway. An oropharyngeal airway is even better if it can be introduced during a period of nonseizure activity and if the patient will tolerate it. The use of the so-called *jaw-spreaders* is not recommended because they can cause trauma to the mouth, teeth, or gums. While airway control is always appropriate, some authorities believe that hypoxia created in a seizing, nonbreathing patient actually in itself limits the seizure. Oxygen is always indicated, especially postseizure. Suctioning is important and may be required. Drug therapy (IV Valium or Dilantin) is desirable for prolonged or recurrent grand mal seizures. An accurate description of the seizure by the field team may be very helpful to follow-up neurological exams in the hospital. Special attention should be given to unilateral or focal activity.

Your patient is admitted to the neurology service with a tentative diagnosis of "seizure, etiology unknown."

CASE STUDY 7C: MR. M. BRICKER

Your paramedic unit is dispatched to a reported vehicle accident with injuries. At this early morning hour you pull the ambulance into the street and are immediately enveloped in fog. You estimate visibility to be less than 50 feet.

There is little traffic, and you proceed with caution. As you approach the accident site, you slow down even more until suddenly, out of the fog, you come upon it. On the pavement directly ahead of you lies a still, human form and next to it a crumpled motorcycle. An accompanying fire department engine company immediately lays out flares to protect the scene. When you reach the patient, you find a male in his early 20s. He is conscious but disoriented and does not remember what happened. He was apparently not wearing a helmet, and your partner finds a large laceration on the patient's right parietal area. There is also an open fracture of the right femur. Your partner continues his examination: pupils are equal and reactive. The patient has no cervical pain, and he moves all extremities. His abdomen is soft, and breath sounds are bilaterally clear. He does have bilateral ecchymosis around both eyes and multiple abrasions to his face, shoulder, and arms. As you make an initial radio report to the hospital, your partner applies a traction splint, cervical collar, sandbags, and backboard.

Of the following factors, which concerns you most about this patient:

1. fractured femur
2. laceration
3. bilateral periorbital ecchymosis
4. mental confusion

The fractured femur initially occupies your attention because of the threat of hypovolemia. The presence of "owl eyes" is also important because it indicates that a great deal of force was absorbed and the possibility of skull fracture is increased. A patient with a previous loss of consciousness or mental confusion should be observed carefully. Easily treatable causes of unconsciousness, such as hypoxia, insulin reaction, hypovolemia, and cardiac arrhythmias, must also be ruled out.

Your partner relays initial vital signs to you. Pulse is 100, respirations are 20, and blood pressure is 124/80. The monitor shows a sinus rhythm. With the traction splint in place and adequate precautions to immobilize the spine, the patient is placed on the gurney with a backboard. Oxygen is given by cannula at 6 l, and the hospital orders an IV with lactated Ringer's at 100 ml per hour.

As the gurney is loaded into the ambulance, there is a screeching of tires behind you. You instinctively whirl to see a pair of headlights appear out of the fog about 30 feet away. The vehicle stops just short of the ambulance. The somewhat inebriated driver had driven through the flare pattern diverting traffic around the scene.

The IV is started easily and taped in place. Your patient, however, has become quite lethargic. He responds by opening his eyes when your partner calls his name but then lapses into unconsciousness. A recheck of his eyes reveals a larger pupil on the right side. His breathing, though somewhat shallow, remains regular. The pulse has dropped to 60. You believe that your patient is showing signs of increased intracranial pressure.

What can you do to treat a possible extending head injury:

1. hyperventilate with oxygen
2. change the IV to 5 percent D/W

3. transport "red lights and siren"
4. place the patient in a Trendelenberg

While immediate transport is obviously necessary for this patient, some intracranial pressure may effectively be relieved by hyperventilation with 100 percent oxygen. This blows off carbon dioxide resulting in venous constriction, which in turn increases available intracranial volume. A "reverse" Trendelenberg (or head elevated) position may also be helpful to reduce cerebral venous pooling.

A pillow is slid underneath the head of the backboard, and your partner ventilates the patient while you inform the hospital of the patient's changing status. An update of vital signs shows a pulse of 60, respirations of 24 with assistance, and blood pressure at 130/80. The patient responds only to deep pain stimulus. The hospital agrees that the patient shows signs of increased intracranial pressure and requests an approximate body weight. You estimate your patient to weigh 180 pounds (82 kg), and you are ordered to start Mannitol, 20 gm IV Volutrol over five minutes.

Mannitol is used in head injury patients with signs of increased intracranial pressure because it

1. causes vasoconstriction
2. controls intracranial bleeding
3. draws fluids from brain cells
4. decreases blood pressure

Mannitol is a diuretic that draws fluid by osmotic gradient from the brain and intracellular spaces, thereby reducing cerebral edema. When increased intracranial pressure is due to hemorrhage, however, this drug is contraindicated. Reducing brain volume allows for greater expansion of the hemorrhage. Since a clearcut distinction is rarely possible in the prehospital phase, Mannitol should be used with due caution.

The Mannitol is hung and piggybacked into the IV line. Ventilations are continued at about 24 per minute, and the monitor still shows a borderline bradycardia. The hospital requests another set of vitals, but you are unable to hear the blood pressure owing to road noise in the ambulance.

With increasing intracranial pressure, what might you expect to happen to the blood pressure:

1. an increase in B/P
2. a decrease in B/P
3. narrowing pulse pressure
4. no change

Changes in vital signs are an ominous sign in a head injury. Because the control centers of the vital functions are located in the brain stem, pressure in this area effects changes in pulse rate, respiratory effort, and blood pressure. Blood pressure, when effected, most often increases with an increase in intracranial pressure. A hypotensive patient with a head injury is probably also hypovolemic.

Upon your arrival at the hospital, the patient is whisked into the emergency room, where a neurosurgeon is standing by. The doctor carefully reviews your serial observations of the patient's deteriorating neurological status, then decides to perform an emergency craniotomy. In surgery a large epidural hematoma is discovered.

Discussion

Management of a patient with severe head injury can be frustrating for the prehospital team. Mortality is understandably high; often little treatment can be initiated in the field. Carefully documented neurological changes can be very important to the hospital staff receiving your patient.

High flow oxygen is always indicated, as well as EKG monitoring. An IV to keep open with normal saline or lactated Ringer's should be started as the situation permits. Most authorities agree that D_5W should be avoided with suspected intracranial injury, because it is more likely to contribute to cerebral edema owing to its hypotonicity. The relative value of administering Mannitol or Decadron (Dexamethasone) in the field is still widely debated. Mannitol, while relatively fast acting, has a reported "rebound" effect actually causing an increase in intracranial pressure after an initial decrease. As the sugar molecules pass into the brain cells, the osmotic gradient is reversed. The use of Decadron in the prehospital setting is limited owing to delay of the onset of action for four to six hours. Finally, traumatic head injuries must always be assumed to be accompanied by spinal injury until ruled out by X-rays. Appropriate immobilization of the patient's neck and spine should always be carried out.

Your patient, though managed carefully by the prehospital team, is beyond help and dies three days later in the trauma unit.

CASE STUDY 7D: MR. T. ALEXANDER

Your paramedic unit is dispatched by a report of a man "unable to walk." After quickly checking the wall map of your response area, you and your partner climb into the ambulance. When you turn the ignition key, however, nothing happens. The starter is apparently not getting any power. You try again and still the engine is silent. Flipping the panel switch to "battery 2," you try the key once again. This time the engine roars to life and you breathe a sigh of relief. (Later investigation shows a broken lead wire as the problem.)

Once at the scene, you grab the necessary equipment and walk to the front door of a modest tract home. You are met by an elderly woman, who leads you into the living room, where her husband sits in a large, overstuffed chair. He is conscious, and his eyes follow your partner, but he does not speak. His breathing is normal at a rate of 16. Checking the patient's radial pulse, your partner reports that it is 74 and irregular. The patient appears to understand questions and is aware of his environment. He does, however, seem unable to speak. Questioning the patient's wife, you determine that this is abnormal.

The term which best describes your patient thus far is

1. aphasic
2. dysphagic
3. phonic
4. mute

This patient is most correctly described as aphasic, or unable to speak. While he is technically mute, this latter condition is more commonly associated with hearing impairment.

The EKG monitor is hooked up to the patient and shows atrial fibrillation. His blood pressure is 168/104, and pupils are equal and reactive. His skin is warm and dry. As your partner continues the physical exam, you question the patient's wife. She tells you that following breakfast her husband went to the living room to read a newspaper. Shortly thereafter, she went to check on him and found that he was unable to talk. He also was unable to stand. Her husband, she says, has high blood pressure and also a history of heart disease. Meanwhile, your partner has put the patient on oxygen by nasal cannula and completed the assessment and notes that the patient has right-sided weakness but no apparent loss of sensation. He exhibits some drooping of facial muscles and is drooling slightly. Pupils are equal and reactive.

This information suggests that the patient may have

1. seizure disorder
2. drug overdose
3. cerebrovascular accident
4. vocal cord paralysis

These findings are characteristic of CVA. Although some of the other conditions might cause similar symptoms, CVA is the only one that commonly produces unilateral findings.

After contacting the hospital, you are requested to start an IV with

5 percent dextrose in water and transport as soon as possible. While your partner is starting an IV, the patient's wife brings you a list of his prescribed medications. It includes Inderal, nitroglycerin, Aldomet, Coumadin, and Lanoxin.

Other than Aldomet (an antihypertensive drug), which of these medications may be most significant to this patient's present condition:

1. Inderal
2. nitroglycerin
3. Coumadin
4. Lanoxin

This patient's medical history of high blood pressure and cardiac disease already makes him a high risk for CVA. In addition, he is taking Coumadin, an anticoagulant. This suggests that this patient may be prone to thrombus or embolus, the most common causes of stroke.

With a patent IV, you and your partner are ready to load the patient. With special care, you ease him from his chair and onto the gurney. The resuscitator bottle is placed gently between his legs, and the EKG monitor is strapped on the gurney. His rhythm remains unchanged. Once in the bright sun, your partner tries to shade the patient's eyes with a hand. With a coordinated lift, the gurney slides smoothly into the ambulance. Climbing behind the steering wheel, you buckle the seatbelt and check your lights.

En route to the hospital, you concentrate on traffic conditions. You make a mental note to check the faulty starter problem when you return to the station. Suddenly there is a squeal of tires from the car ahead as it swerves sharply to avoid colliding with a second vehicle pulling from the curb. The two automobiles collide with a loud bang as sheet metal and structural steel collapse in thousandths of a second. Your vehicle fortunately is far enough back to avoid the collision.

Given the following choices, what would you do:

1. notify your dispatcher and continue to the hospital
2. have your partner stay with the patient while you check for injuries
3. stop, render aid, and transport any patients from the vehicle accident
4. stop and set out flares

Mindful that your primary legal obligation is to the patient whom you are already treating, the decision whether to stop at the accident scene may well become a moral one. Depending upon the current condition of your patient, distance to the hospital, availability of responding units, and other variables, you may choose to stop and at least determine the extent of injuries involved. However, it must be underscored that to leave your patient unattended can constitute abandonment, for which you could be held liable.

You decide to stop and determine if anyone is seriously injured. While your partner remains with your patient, you quickly examine the drivers of the two autos. Their injuries are minor, and, after explaining that more help is on the way, you continue to the hospital.

Discussion

Cerebrovascular accidents are seen most frequently in elderly patients. Often they may have predisposing factors such as hypertension, heart disease, atherosclerosis, emboli or thrombi, anticoagulant therapy, intracranial lesions or tumors, and aneurysms. Signs and symptoms may include altered levels of consciousness, speech disorders (from slurred to aphasic), incontinence, drooling, facial drooping, unilateral paralysis, or marked weakness. Occasionally, pupils may be unequal. Similar to CVAs are transient ischemic attacks (TIA) in which signs and symptoms are only temporary, many times resolving before the arrival of the prehospital care team.

Treatment of a CVA patient is relatively basic. Airway control is of prime importance and should be appropriately managed. Oxygen should be administered, and suctioning may be necessary. An IV line to keep open can be started, depending on the patient's condition. A careful history and complete physical exam will be extremely helpful, with special attention made to neurologic status. Any neurologic dysfunction should be carefully recorded. It should also be kept in mind that hypoglycemia can mimic many of the signs of CVA. Therefore, 50 percent glucose should be considered, especially for patients with an altered level of consciousness.

Your patient has, in fact, suffered a stroke. He makes good progress, however, and is discharged home for convalescing after one week in the hospital.

RELATED ASSESSMENT QUESTIONS

7.1 The dosage of Valium for control of active or prolonged seizure is
- **(a)** 0.5–2 mg slow IV push
- **(b)** 2.5–40 mg IV push, titrated to effect
- **(c)** 5–20 mg in 500 ml IV drip
- **(d)** 25–50 mg deep IM
- **(e)** 100 mg in 50 ml IV Volutrol, over 20 minutes

7.2 Which of the following best describes the philosophy of airway maintenance for a suspected spinal cord injury:
- **(a)** the cord injury takes precedence over airway; the patient can be ventilated only if it can be done without moving anything.
- **(b)** the airway takes precedence over the cord; the airway must be opened regardless of whatever damage it might do to the cord

(c) there is no difference in management; in the presence of cord injury the airway is still opened in the usual way
(d) special techniques must be employed to open the airway without moving the cord
(e) it is unnecessary to take any special precautions, because the cord can't be damaged simply by opening the airway

7.3 Which of the following statements about a person with Cheyne-Stokes respirations is *true:*
(a) the patient is breathing in the normal, healthy mode and should be left alone
(b) the patient is breathing in an abnormal pattern with inadequate exchange and should be assisted
(c) the patient is apneic and needs immediate resuscitation
(d) the patient is hyperventilating and should breathe into a paper bag
(e) the patient is breathing abnormally but does not require any assistance

7.4 Which of the following is not included in the *routine* management of a patient with CVA:
(a) suctioning
(b) IV fluid replacement
(c) oxygen
(d) positioning
(e) EKG monitoring

7.5 Which of the following is *least* likely to be an early sign of increased intracranial pressure:
(a) depressed level of consciousness
(b) hypotension
(c) bradycardia
(d) abnormal respiratory patterns
(e) pupil changes

7.6 Which of the following is *least* important in assessing neurological status:
(a) does the patient respond to voice stimuli?
(b) are the pupils equal and reactive to light?
(c) does the patient have deep tendon reflexes?
(d) are the hand grasps equal and normal in strength?
(e) is the patient able to move all extremities?

7.7 Spinal cord injury should be suspected in any patient who presents with
(a) head injury
(b) facial injury
(c) multiple trauma
(d) unconsciousness following trauma
(e) any of the above

7.8 Which of the following is *least* likely to be included in the treatment of spinal cord injury:
(a) vasopressors
(b) analgesics
(c) antishock trousers
(d) positive pressure ventilator
(e) IV normal saline

7.9 Which of the following is *least* effective in assessing the level of consciousness:
(a) response to voice
(b) orientation to surroundings
(c) response to pain
(d) ability to move extremities
(e) response to touch

7.10 You were called to the home of a 50-year-old female who is lying on the couch. She is having trouble explaining why she called. Her speech is slurred, and she can't seem to find the right words to use. As you examine her, you find that her hand grasps are unequal, and her face seems droopy on one side. She is drooling slightly and is unable to sit up without help. You suspect that she
(a) is having an MI
(b) has had a CVA
(c) needs a pacemaker
(d) has muscular dystrophy
(e) is intoxicated or under the influence of drugs

7.11 In which of the following situations would it be appropriate to administer Valium:
(a) a diagnosed epileptic who is in a postictal state
(b) a child who experienced febrile convulsions
(c) a woman with toxemia of pregnancy who had a grand mal seizure but remained oxygenated throughout the episode
(d) a man who is having recurrent prolonged seizures of unknown etiology
(e) all of the above

7.12 Which of the following is the most important side effect of Valium when it is administered IV:
(a) loss of consciousness
(b) hypertension
(c) respiratory depression/arrest
(d) idiopathic ventricular standstill
(e) sustained seizure activity

7.13 Which of the following would be the most appropriate reason for ammonia ampules:
- **(a)** to augment nitroglycerin in treating angina
- **(b)** to terminate a syncopal episode
- **(c)** to revive a patient in Stokes-Adams
- **(d)** to stimulate respirations in narcotic overdose
- **(e)** to clean the ambulance after transporting a tuberculosis patient

7.14 Mannitol is administered to patients with head injury who exhibit
- **(a)** unconsciousness
- **(b)** signs of increased intracranial pressure
- **(c)** life-threatening cardiac arrhythmias
- **(d)** drop in blood pressure
- **(e)** increase in pulse rate

7.15 In a patient with a cervical injury, the airway can *best* be opened by
- **(a)** hyperextending the neck
- **(b)** turning the head to one side
- **(c)** ventilating with the neck flexed
- **(d)** pulling the jaw upward
- **(e)** performing a tracheostomy

7.16 Which of the following best explains why analgesics are contraindicated in head injury and trauma situations:
- **(a)** they suppress the level of consciousness
- **(b)** they can mask symptoms
- **(c)** they can cause hypotension
- **(d)** they hinder assessment
- **(e)** all of the above

7.17 Which of the following statements about Mannitol is *not* true:
- **(a)** it is a cerebral diuretic
- **(b)** it can cause renal failure
- **(c)** the usual dosage is 2 gm IV Volutrol over five minutes
- **(d)** the solution has a tendency to crystalize in the bottle/bag
- **(e)** it requires administration through an in-line filter

7.18 Which of the following contraindicates the use of Mannitol:
- **(a)** head trauma
- **(b)** seizures
- **(c)** suspected intracranial bleeding
- **(d)** spinal cord trauma
- **(e)** increased intracranial pressure

7.19 Your patient is lethargic and confused and can't remember the immediate past, yawns frequently, and keeps drifting off to sleep. You should suspect
- **(a)** CVA
- **(b)** atropine toxicity

(c) postictal state
(d) nitrogen narcosis
(e) hyperventilation syndrome

7.20 Continuous grand mal seizures are treated with all of the following *except*
(a) protection from injury
(b) high flow oxygen
(c) IV Valium titrated to effect
(d) physical restraints
(e) suctioning as needed

7.21 Which of the following physical signs does *not* suggest skull fracture:
(a) clear drainage from ear
(b) black and blue marks around eyes
(c) red "mask" across nose
(d) ecchymosis behind ears
(e) palpable deformity

7.22 When caring for a patient with head injury, you should anticipate and monitor fluctuations in all of the following *except*
(a) sensorium
(b) muscle tone
(c) vital signs
(d) respiratory status
(e) pupils

ANSWER KEY

7.1 b	**7.7** e	**7.13** b	**7.18** c
7.2 d	**7.8** b	**7.14** b	**7.19** c
7.3 b	**7.9** d	**7.15** d	**7.20** d
7.4 b	**7.10** b	**7.16** e	**7.21** c
7.5 b	**7.11** d	**7.17** c	**7.22** b
7.6 c	**7.12** c		

8

SOFT TISSUE INJURIES

CASE STUDY 8A: MR. G. FORDE

Your paramedic ambulance and a fire department engine company respond to a report of an auto versus telephone pole. As you round a blind curve, the night sky is illuminated by an eerie orange glow. You can see it: The car is on fire. You and your partner quickly don protective clothing as firefighters stretch a hoseline from the pumper to the burning auto. Flames engulf the entire front end of the crumpled vehicle, illuminating a darkened form slumped over the steering wheel. The hose nozzle is opened; as the spray sweeps across the flames, the fire is rapidly extinguished.

Miraculously the driver's door opens normally as steam rises from the still hot metal. Inside the car is a male, unconscious but alive. He is removed from the wreckage on a backboard and loaded into the ambulance. With the adequate lighting, you begin a systematic head-to-toe exam. Your patient is in his late 40s and unconscious. You carefully remove his clothing in order to check for further injuries. Part of the shirt-sleeve is embedded in the wound and left in place. Your partner puts him on oxygen at 8 l by mask. The patient has an obvious fracture of his left femur. There are second- and some third-degree burns to portions of his upper torso, arms, neck, and face. Appropriate treatment of this patient should include all of the following except

1. IV Ringer's lactate or normal saline
2. morphine sulfate, up to 10 mg IV

3. sterile burn sheet
4. Hare traction splint

Morphine, while used extensively as an analgesic in burn victims, is not indicated for this unconscious patient. It is important to observe closely any neurological deficit or changes in a patient with an altered level of consciousness.

Using the "Rule of Nines" as a guide, you estimate the extent of burns in this man to be about 30 percent second-degree and 10 percent third-degree (40 percent of total body area). Vital signs are pulse 110, respirations 28, and B/P 152/80. The EKG monitor shows a sinus tachycardia. Listening to lung sounds, you hear wheezes on both sides. The traction splint and burn sheet are applied. Because of severe burns on the patient's arms, you decide to start the IV in his uninjured leg. Your management of a severe burn is primarily aimed at controlling which of the following complications:

1. infection
2. kidney failure
3. pulmonary edema
4. hypovolemia

Given the total area and extent of burns in this patient, fluid replacement is essential to combat hypovolemia. As disrupted capillary beds continue to ooze plasma, fluid loss in the first 24 hours postburn can be dramatic. Though seldom seen in the prehospital phase, pulmonary edema secondary to a respiratory burn should also be kept in mind. In this patient, the presence of facial burns, burns that occurred in a confined space, and wheezing suggest a high probability of some respiratory involvement.

The patient begins to regain consciousness en route to the emergency room. He is conscious but confused and is oriented only to his name. You examine his pupils: They are equal and reactive. There is no obvious head trauma. What might you suspect as the cause for this patient's previous loss of consciousness:

1. carbon monoxide poisoning
2. alcohol intoxication
3. hypoglycemia
4. cardiac arrhythmia

Obviously, any of these can induce a loss of consciousness. Smoke inhalation specifically induces a decreased level of consciousness, as carbon monoxide readily combines with hemoglobin, producing a hypoxic effect on the brain. This can be reversed in most cases by using 100 percent oxygen at high flow rates.

Upon arrival at the hospital, you find the emergency room a flurry of activity. The physician and the staff are working on a patient in cardiac arrest, and a single nurse briefly breaks away to instruct you as to a bed for your patient. As you transfer him to the bed, you are dispatched to another incident.

When you return to the hospital for a follow-up, you are confronted by an angry head nurse. The nurse is upset and tells you that too much time was spent at the scene with the burn patient and that your estimation of the area of burn was, in her opinion, "completely wrong." She refuses to listen to anything that you have to say and abruptly walks away. You decide to handle this situation by

1. ignoring the whole thing
2. asking the ED doctor for his opinion
3. discussing the incident with her at a later time
4. insisting that she hear your side

Professionals who work together under stressful conditions will inevitably have an occasional conflict. It is usually most constructive to allow some time to elapse in order to regain a proper perspective. True communication takes place only when our thoughts are successfully understood by the person with whom we are communicating. This cannot be fostered in an atmosphere of anger and misunderstanding.

After your shift you and your partner decide to drop by the emergency room in order to talk with the nurse about the run. It is a quiet morning as the three of you sit in the deserted staff lounge over a cup of coffee. Unlike the pressurized atmosphere of the night before, it is now much easier to explain your feelings, with objectivity restored. Her concern was primarily one of too much time spent on the scene with this critically burned patient. You assure her that it was clear to you that a prompt transport was necessary. Hearing additional information from you about the incident soon convinces her that you performed your assessment and treatment as rapidly as possible under the circumstances.

CASE STUDY 8B: STANLEY R.

"Lifeline 1, respond to child with an eye injury . . . 1746 White Horse Drive, map page 22, B4." You and your partner, just starting your evening meal, head for the squad truck. Dinner will have to wait. Traffic is moderate, and your partner shuts down the siren as you turn into the residential area. A teenage girl frantically waves at you from the curb in front of the address you were given.

"It's my brother," she tells you hurriedly. "He's been shot in the eye with a BB gun."

She leads you into the backyard. Sitting on a deck chair is a young boy, perhaps 10 years old. He is whimpering and cupping both hands to his right eye. As your partner gently begins to check the patient, you attempt to get additional information from the girl. The boy's name is Stanley; they were playing in the yard with a BB rifle when it discharged into the boy's eye at close range. She was supposed to be babysitting her brother and is very upset. The parents, you discover, have gone out for dinner, and she doesn't know how to reach them.

Meanwhile, your partner has coaxed the young boy to remove his hands in order to get a good look at the eye. Using a penlight, you both can see the wound. There is a small, 5–6 mm laceration at the four o'clock position on the sclera. The cornea is clear and the pupil responds normally. A trace of clear, gelatinous material is also visible, oozing from the wound.

You could appropriately assume that this material is

1. foreign matter
2. corneal fragments
3. lacrimal secretions
4. vitreous humor

Behind the lens lies the vitreous body, a gelatinous mass that fills the globe of the eye. Direct penetration through the sclera (white portion of the eye) into this cavity may cause leakage of the vitreous humor, which has a poor prognosis.

The patient complains of an intense burning sensation in the injured eye. In addition, he describes visual disturbances, including intermittent blindness with occasional flashes of bright light. Vision in his left eye is normal. Vital signs are also normal, and there are no other apparent injuries. With great care your partner places eye patches on both eyes and gently tapes them in place.

Covering both eyes with dressings is recommended because

1. it is difficult to bandage one eye only
2. it helps prevent sympathetic movement of the injured eye
3. it decreases the patient's awareness of the injured eye
4. it makes the patient more dependent upon the EMT

Application of sterile dressings to both eyes is utilized primarily to prevent sympathetic movement of the injured eye in unison with the normal eye.

This is especially important with severe eye injuries, as here. Additionally, foreign bodies in the eye may cause secondary injury should the eye or eyelids be subjected to unnecessary movement.

After a quick secondary exam, the boy is taken to the waiting ambulance. Your partner climbs aboard, and you follow with the squad.

Transporting this minor to a medical facility without parental consent is

1. legally acceptable in emergency situations
2. unlawful without prior court approval
3. lawful if accompanied by a peace officer
4. unlawful and constitutes kidnapping

The law properly assumes that transport of a minor to a medical facility by EMTs in the absence of the parents is acceptable in emergency situations. Under such circumstances, consent is implied. Once at the emergency department, however, treatment of a minor is limited to bona fide parental consent or approval of the court (a procedure that may be performed by phone in a very brief time).

Once at the hospital, an eye specialist is waiting for your young patient. X-ray studies show the BB inside the eyeball. Fortunately it is in one piece and, though delicate, can be surgically removed. In addition, the ophthalmologist believes that the injury has caused a detached retina, which must also be repaired. The patient is prepped for surgery later that evening.

Injuries to the eye must always be treated with extreme care. While prehospital treatment is limited, several points should be reviewed.

Caustic Agents

Whenever caustic agents (acids, alkalis, petroleum distillates, etc.) come in contact with the eye, the eye must be flushed thoroughly with large amounts of water. Sterile saline is ideal as an irrigating solution and is less likely to cause additional discomfort. Continuous irrigation over a 10-minute period is recommended (20 minutes if the caustic agent is an alkali).

Foreign Bodies

Foreign bodies in the eye, if detected, may be removed with an irrigating solution. If a foreign body is not visible on the surface of the eye, it may be adhering to the upper or lower eyelid. The upper lid can be gently everted by rolling it over a cotton-tipped applicator, thereby exposing the undersurface. The foreign body can then be removed with another moist, sterile swab. A foreign body on the surface of the eye and resistant to irrigation should not be removed in the field. Obviously, the examiner's hands should be thoroughly cleansed before attempting any treatment. Because the presence of a foreign body may also produce a minor abrasion to the corneal surface, further examination in the emergency department is recommended.

Penetrating Injuries

A penetrating injury to the eye is severe indeed. If there is an impaled object, no attempt should be made to remove it. Instead, the eye should be covered with a protective cone (disposable drinking cup, etc.) and a loose dressing applied. Lacerations to the eye should be treated by covering both eyes with a loose protective dressing. No external pressure should be applied.

Topical ointments and solutions (other than irrigating solutions) are contraindicated in the field. Visual disturbances such as blurred or double vision, loss of sight, or other aberrations should be recorded.

Despite delicate microsurgery, your young patient's traumatized eye does not respond; there is permanent loss of sight to that eye.

RELATED ASSESSMENT QUESTIONS

8.1 Your patient is a male, 22-year-old college student who complains of abdominal pain following a rough tackle during a football game. He has his knees drawn up toward his chest; inspection of the abdomen shows marked distension and some rigidity. His skin is pale and clammy. His blood pressure is 102/68, pulse is 132, and respirations are 22. Your actions should include

- **(a)** auscultation of bowel sounds, antishock trousers, and an IV of 5 percent D/W
- **(b)** an IV of RL to maintain blood pressure, oxygen, and rapid transport
- **(c)** morphine sulfate, oxygen, and an IV TKO
- **(d)** oxygen, dopamine, and prompt transport
- **(e)** further assessment of the abdomen, antishock trousers, and morphine

8.2 Which of the following is contraindicated in the treatment of frostbite:

- **(a)** gentle rewarming
- **(b)** dry wraps
- **(c)** protection of blistered areas
- **(d)** gentle rubbing with snow
- **(e)** protection from recooling

8.3 Which of the following would *not* be appropriate for a patient who has major second- and third-degree burns:

- **(a)** oxygen
- **(b)** morphine

(c) antibiotic ointments
(d) IV Ringer's lactate
(e) clean dressings

8.4 Treatment of electrical burns should include all of the following *except*
(a) monitoring EKG
(b) starting an IV
(c) administering high flow oxygen
(d) flushing a burn with copious amounts of water
(e) application of sterile dressings

8.5 A patient found unconscious at the scene of a fire should be suspected of having
(a) diabetes
(b) third-degree burns
(c) respiratory burns
(d) carbon monoxide poisoning
(e) drug overdose

8.6 Your *first* concern with a burn patient is
(a) estimation of the extent of the burn
(b) determination of the degree of the burn
(c) identification of the source of the burn
(d) evaluation of the airway
(e) assessment of vital signs and EKG

8.7 Which of the following is *least* important in determining the severity of the burn injury:
(a) depth
(b) extent
(c) involvement of critical areas
(d) age of patient
(e) level of consciousness

8.8 The "Rule of Nines" applies to
(a) children with abdominal trauma
(b) children with fractures
(c) adults with burns
(d) anybody with burns
(e) anybody with abdominal trauma

8.9 The earliest threat from a severe burn is
(a) infection
(b) renal failure
(c) pulmonary embolus
(d) loss of consciousness
(e) shock

8.10 Initial treatment of a chemical burn is to
(a) apply a weak vinegar solution

(b) give sodium bicarbonate IV
(c) sponge with hydrogen peroxide
(d) flush with water
(e) give specific antidote for the chemical

8.11 Abdominal evisceration should be treated by all of the following *except*
(a) withholding analgesics and oral fluids
(b) replacing the protruding organ
(c) covering the wound with damp sterile dressing
(d) administering oxygen
(e) starting an IV of RL or NS

8.12 Which of the following positions is *least* acceptable for transporting a patient with facial trauma:
(a) on the patient's back, head down
(b) on the patient's side, head level
(c) on the patient's side, head up
(d) on the patient's stomach, head up
(e) on the patient's stomach, head level

8.13 Which of the following is *not* an effective method of removing foreign particles from the eye:
(a) flush with saline
(b) rub the closed eye
(c) invert the eyelid
(d) use a corner of a gauze pad
(e) natural lacrimation

8.14 The greatest threat from facial injuries is
(a) blood loss
(b) airway obstruction
(c) loss of vision
(d) disfiguration
(e) extreme pain

8.15 Your patient has a fractured mandible. You have controlled bleeding and immobilized the jaw by aligning teeth and applying a bandage. Which of the following factors causes you greatest concern:
(a) the patient's jaw hurts
(b) the patient can't talk
(c) the patient's respiratory rate is 24
(d) the patient complains of headache
(e) the patient complains of nausea

8.16 Control of bleeding associated with epistaxis is usually accomplished by
(a) use of a hemostat
(b) direct pressure at the pressure point
(c) application of ice

(d) application of a tourniquet
(e) pinching of the nostrils

ANSWER KEY

8.1 b	**8.5** d	**8.9** e	**8.13** b
8.2 d	**8.6** d	**8.10** d	**8.14** b
8.3 c	**8.7** e	**8.11** b	**8.15** e
8.4 d	**8.8** c	**8.12** a	**8.16** e

9

MUSCULOSKELETAL AND MULTISYSTEM TRAUMA

CASE STUDY 9A: MR. A. RODERIKO

You are dispatched to a call for a man who has fallen from a roof. You recognize the address as being on a new street just added to your mapbook the week before. A brief four-minute response brings you into an area where a housing tract is being constructed, and there are few visible addresses. Fortunately, a worker waves your ambulance to the curb. You and your partner are directed behind a two-story house, where you find your patient lying on the ground. He is a 36-year-old male who is conscious and has an open fracture on his left femur. He tells you that he was working on the roof when he lost his footing and fell backward, landing on hard-packed dirt. Looking up, you estimate the distance to the roof to be about 18 to 20 feet. The patient tells you that he remembers the fall and seems to be oriented. He has no neck pain but hurts when you palpate the lumbar region. His skin is warm and moist, and his pupils are equal and reactive. There is deformity in his left elbow, and he complains of severe pain in his fractured leg.

Of the following choices, which would be the most appropriate to splint this lower extremity

1. cardboard splint
2. full-leg splint
3. traction splint
4. ladder splint

While splinting depends upon available equipment and individual technique, the most appropriate immobilization of a femoral shaft fracture is a traction splint. Application of this device provides traction against the powerful quadriceps muscle in the thigh, reducing the possibility of secondary damage to muscle tissue, nerves, and blood vessels. While some controversy exists regarding whether exposed bone ends should be allowed to reenter the wound when traction is applied, surgical intervention will be required, regardless, in the reduction and repair of this fracture. Therefore, surgical debridement and prophylactic use of antibiotics will take care of any bacteria introduced in this manner.

Next you check the patient's vital signs: His pulse is 92, respirations are 18, and blood pressure is 118/70. While you adjust the traction splint for proper length, your partner applies a cervical collar as a normal precaution. Before applying the splint to the leg, you check for a palpable pulse on the top of his left foot; there is none. There is, however, no apparent loss of sensation.

How else might you check for vascular impairment in this fractured limb:

1. bilateral capillary refilling time
2. presence of a posterior tibial pulse
3. distal skin color and temperature
4. all of the above

The absence of a pulse and/or loss of sensation distal to a fracture site are of significant concern with any orthopedic injury. With a fractured lower extremity, the absence of a dorsalis pedis pulse is in itself not conclusive of vascular impairment; few people normally have this condition. In this event, other signs, such as those mentioned, should be examined.

Upon examination you find that your patient's foot is cool and pale and that there is a lag in capillary refilling on the affected limb. As gentle traction is applied, however, the posterior tibial pulse becomes weakly palpable, and the foot begins to return to normal color. A sterile dressing is placed over the open wound, and the traction splint is quickly applied. You note that the patient also has some relief from the pain of the injury. A well-padded pair of ladder splints is used to immobilize his possibly dislocated elbow. Your patient continues to complain of some lower back pain as well; an aluminum scoop stretcher is placed underneath him, and he is transferred to the gurney. In the ambulance, radio contact is made with the hospital. After an initial assessment is relayed, you are instructed to start an intravenous line.

Which of the following is the best reason to start a volume expanding IV solution in this patient:

1. he will require an IV before going to surgery
2. he is showing signs of shock

3. he may have internal injuries
4. a fractured femur can involve significant blood loss

Hypovolemia secondary to a fractured femur is not uncommon. In fact, up to a liter of whole blood can be sequestered in the tissues surrounding this bone in a very short time. While this patient may have internal injuries that are as yet covert, the presence of this obvious fracture is significant enough to warrant an IV with normal saline, lactated Ringer's, or some similar isotonic solution.

An IV of normal saline is started with a large-bore cannula in the patient's right arm. After hooking him up to the EKG monitor, you observe normal sinus rhythm. In the ambulance, you complete the physical exam. There is no evidence of chest injury, and lung sounds are clear upon auscultation. The abdomen is negative; however, the patient does complain of pain when you stress the iliac crests bilaterally. The audible systole "beep" of the cardiac monitor suddenly draws your attention as the patient's pulse rate has increased to 130. His skin has become cool and moist, and the blood pressure is 92/60. Your partner opens the IV to wide-open and immediately notifies the hospital of the patient's deteriorating condition. You are requested to apply antishock trousers stat.

With the traction splint already in place, which of the following options would you now choose in applying the antishock trousers:

1. remove the traction splint and apply the antishock suit
2. suggest that a second IV be started
3. refuse to apply the antishock trousers due to a possible fractured pelvis
4. apply the antishock trousers and inflate one leg and abdominal compartments only

Although the presence of a traction splint presents a minor complication when used with the antishock trousers, it does not prevent the application of this device over it. Inflation of the shock suit should, however, be limited to the unaffected leg and abdominal compartment except in cases of severe hypotension.

With some difficulty, the antishock trousers are slid underneath the patient and inflated. Your patient complains of pain as the abdominal section is pumped up; full inflation of that compartment is not achieved. The blood pressure is 106/0 by palpation. The IV continues to run wide open. In addition, oxygen has been started at 8 l by cannula. Within a few minutes the ambulance pulls up to the emergency room. Hospital staff are standing by to escort you and your patient into the treatment area as you unload the gurney. A nurse takes a new set of vital signs, which appear within normal limits.

As your partner briefs the attending physician, another nurse disconnects the pump from the antishock trousers and quickly opens a valve to deflate the leg compartment. Almost simultaneously you and your partner, realizing the potential danger of rapidly deflating the device, reach for the open valve to shut off the escaping air. Later you find that this nurse had been sent down from a medical floor to "cover" for a regular ER nurse on sick leave and was unfamiliar with the application and use of the antishock trousers. After initial X-rays in the emergency room, your patient is found to have a fractured femur and a dislocated elbow. An abdominal lavage is performed but is negative for intraabdominal bleeding; however, in surgery, gross blood is discovered in the retroperitoneal area as a result of a fractured pelvis.

Discussion

Orthopedic injuries are generally treated in a low-key fashion in the field, which is often appropriate. Early assessment of possible vascular impairment and attention to proper immobilization of the injured area are a priority. Since considerable force is required to break an adult bone, this fact should be considered when examining the patient for associated injuries. It is equally important to observe the scene for evidence of a mechanism of injury that may be helpful in determining the relative force encountered to produce such an injury. Injury to the neck and spine must always be assumed in cases of multiple trauma and appropriate precautions taken (i.e., cervical collar, backboard, and sandbags). Since the major field complication with fractures will be hypovolemia, the judicious use of intravenous fluids and other antishock measures should be considered and instituted as necesssary. Patients who require surgical reduction of their injury should also be considered for an IV even though hypovolemia may not pose an immediate problem.

Your 36-year-old patient responds well in surgery and in 10 weeks is participating in a rehabilitative physical therapy program as an outpatient.

CASE STUDY 9B: MR. E. NICHOLAS

Your paramedic ambulance is dispatched to meet with police units at a temporary command post on a downtown street. As you approach the area, you are stopped at a barricade that cordons off two city blocks. You are told that there has been an armed robbery of a local bank and prompt action by police has trapped two robbers inside with six hostages. A SWAT (special weapons and tactics) team is in charge of the operation, and your unit has been requested to stand by. As you park the vehicle, you gaze down the street at a scene that could be right out of a television police show. Being there, however, quickly dissolves images of Hollywood as an involuntary shudder sweeps down your spine.

Suddenly there is a burst of gunfire and the sound reverberates against the multistory buildings lining each side of the street. Almost as immediate is the silence that follows. A pungent odor of gunsmoke surrounds you. Moments later a SWAT team member, dressed in his dark blue combat outfit, escorts your partner and you to the bank. All of the hostages, two men and four women, are unhurt, he tells you. One of the robbers is unhurt and in custody but the other has suffered multiple gunshot wounds. As you enter the bank, you find shattered glass across the lobby. Bank employees are clustered in one corner, being interviewed by police.

Behind the tellers' counter you find the second suspect. He is a male in his late 20s. He is conscious and groaning, his hands clutching his abdomen. Pulling up his bloodstained shirt, you see two separate wounds. One is in the right lower quadrant, and the other is near the right midaxillary line at the rib margin. You estimate the external blood loss to be about 300 to 400 mls. There is only a small amount of active bleeding, and sterile 4-by-4 dressings are applied over the wounds. Oxygen is started by mask at 6l, and your partner hangs an IV set.

Which of the following would you do prior to transport:

1. start the IV
2. obtain vital signs
3. check pupils
4. palpate the abdomen

A well-organized approach to patient assessment is essential to proper management of any medical emergency. In trauma cases, time spent at the scene should be kept to a minimum. In this case, vital signs would be the most important information to obtain prior to transporting.

Vital signs reveal that your patient's blood pressure is 112/82, pulse is 120, and respirations are 28 and shallow. His skin is warm and moist. Lung sounds are clear to auscultation on the left side but seem to be decreased on the right. The patient appears to be alert but refuses to talk to you. He is obviously in a lot of pain as he continues to groan and draw his knees up toward his abdomen. Your partner has started an IV with lactated Ringer's.

Which of the following crucial information has been conspicuously absent from the findings thus far:

1. exit wounds
2. extremity movement
3. pupil size and reactivity
4. tracheal shift

Entrance and exit wounds can be difficult to differentiate, depending upon the size and type of bullet. Generally, entrance wounds are smaller punctures or lacerations due to the relative high velocity of the bullet as it enters the body and little change in shape (i.e., mushrooming, fragmentation, etc.) of the projectile. Exit wounds can be larger and may even appear as an avulsion. Often wounds, whether entrance or exit, are missed on the posterior side of the patient. Turning your patient on his side, you see a single exit wound approximately 4 cm to the right of the spine in the lower thoracic area.

Despite rapid assessment and treatment, when you recheck vital signs the blood pressure is 80/60, pulse is 140, and respirations are 36 and increasingly labored. Your patient's condition is deteriorating. Your partner requests an order for antishock trousers from the hospital, and it is given. Additionally, you are authorized to start another IV to maintain the blood pressure at 100 systolic. Before inflating the antishock trousers, however, something instinctively tells you to pause. Quickly surveying your shocky patient, you see prominent neck vein distention. Auscultating breath sounds show them to be completely absent on the right side. The patient is also cool and very diaphoretic.

With this new information, you should

1. inflate the antishock trousers immediately
2. administer positive pressure ventilation
3. request an order for needle thoracostomy
4. prepare for immediate transport

Depending upon your training and protocols, you should select either answer 1 or 2. This patient has probably developed a tension pneumothorax, compromising right heart return, as indicated by the distended neck veins. Such shock symptoms along with significant neck vein distention are not due to hypovolemia despite the fact that this patient has had traumatic abdominal injury. Inflation of the antishock trousers and additional IV fluids will only contribute to the patient's rapid deterioration. Definitive therapy for tension pneumothorax is thoracic decompression by needle thoracostomy or insertion of a chest tube. If it is not possible to perform this procedure in the field, immediate transport is indicated.

Because you are not permitted to perform either of these procedures, you must transport now. The nearest emergency department is about six minutes away. Hospital staff are standing by when you arrive with your semiconscious patient. After quickly evaluating his condition, the physician orders a chest tray set up and then inserts the trocar on the right midaxillary line. A wisp of escaping air confirms the decompression of a tension pneumothorax. ABGs, portable chest X-ray, CBC, type and crossmatch, and Foley catheter are also ordered.

Discussion

Gunshot wounds can vary from simple grazes to serious intraabdominal, intrathoracic, or intracranial injuries. Frequently, trauma of this type will require surgical intervention for patient survival. Early contact with the receiving hospital is advisable in order to avoid unnecessary delay activating an operating room (OR) team. Field treatment is generally limited to support of cardiovascular and ventilatory status. Rapid assessment and transport should receive highest priority. Any incident involving a gunshot wound, accidental or otherwise, will require investigation by a law enforcement agency. Your initial observations on the scene may be used later in a criminal case.

Unlike other penetrating injuries of relatively low velocity, such as a stabbing, a gunshot wound represents far greater potential for tissue destruction, because its energy is rapidly absorbed. Even the presence of an entry and exit wound does not guarantee a straight-line path of the bullet. Fragmentation of the bullet or ricochet of the projectile may produce damage to organs and other tissues not anatomically adjacent to the apparent path of the bullet.

Your patient undergoes surgery for his injuries and later recovers to face criminal charges.

RELATED ASSESSMENT QUESTIONS

9.1 Fracture of the femur is considered dangerous in the field because of the threat of
- **(a)** permanent disability
- **(b)** loss of consciousness
- **(c)** hypovolemic shock
- **(d)** extreme pain and subsequent hyperventilation
- **(e)** neurogenic shock

9.2 Upon examination you find that your multiple trauma patient has significant abdominal rigidity. This is most specifically suggestive of
- **(a)** shock
- **(b)** aneurysm
- **(c)** internal bleeding
- **(d)** appendicitis
- **(e)** perforated bowel

9.3 Which of the following is *not* included in the treatment of open fractures:
- **(a)** control bleeding and dress wound
- **(b)** immobilize extremity
- **(c)** start an IV to replace fluids
- **(d)** give small doses of analgesics as needed
- **(e)** evaluate pulses and sensation distal to the injury

9.4 An isolated femoral fracture should be treated with all of the following *except*
- **(a)** a traction splint
- **(b)** control of any external bleeding

(c) IV for volume replacement
(d) evaluation of peripheral pulses
(e) immobilization of both legs

9.5 Which of the following poses the greatest potential for hypovolemic shock:
(a) dislocated shoulder
(b) fractured pelvis
(c) fractured tibia/fibula
(d) fractured humerous
(e) sprained ankle

9.6 Which of the following is *not* appropriate for assessing peripheral nerve integrity distal to a musculoskeletal injury:
(a) ask the patient to move fingers/toes
(b) use pinpricks
(c) check for capillary refill
(d) ask about feeling in fingers/toes
(e) all of the above are appropriate

9.7 A traction splint is used to immobilize
(a) sprained fingers
(b) broken ankles
(c) fractured femurs
(d) dislocated elbows
(e) broken arms

9.8 Management of a patient with musculoskeletal trauma will include all of the following *except*
(a) high flow oxygen
(b) IV for possible volume replacement
(c) antishock measures
(d) immobilization
(e) MS in small increments for pain

9.9 A dislocated hip should be treated by all of the following *except*
(a) strong traction to replace the joint
(b) immobilization of both legs
(c) oxygen, IV, and prompt transport
(d) close check on blood pressure and pulse
(e) antishock measures

9.10 Circulation distal to a musculoskeletal injury is best assessed by
(a) asking the patient to move fingers/toes
(b) using pinpricks
(c) checking blood pressure
(d) palpating peripheral pulses
(e) all of the above

9.11 Examination reveals that your patient has a fractured mandible, arterial bleeding from a leg wound, a compound fracture of the left arm, and severe difficulty breathing. What would you do first:
(a) set the fractured mandible
(b) check for airway obstruction
(c) control arterial bleeding
(d) give oxygen by positive pressure
(e) contact the hospital

9.12 You have controlled the bleeding in your multiple trauma patient and have started replacing lost fluids with Ringer's lactate. The patient continues to complain of pain. You listen to the patient's chest and detect rales. You should
(a) give Aminophylline
(b) have the patient sit up
(c) give morphine
(d) slow down the IV
(e) apply antishock trousers

9.13 Your multiple trauma patient is hypotensive from blood loss. You have given 500 ml of RL and have another 500 ml running wide open, but the shock state persists. You might now consider all of the following *except*
(a) antishock trousers
(b) an additional IV line
(c) calcium chloride
(d) plasma volume expanders
(e) immediate transport

ANSWER KEY

9.1 c
9.2 c
9.3 d
9.4 e
9.5 b
9.6 c
9.7 c
9.8 e
9.9 a
9.10 d
9.11 b
9.12 d
9.13 c

10

GENERAL MEDICAL EMERGENCIES

CASE STUDY 10A: MR. S. MARINO

Your paramedic unit responds to a report of a hiker who has been bitten by a snake. Your pickup location is given as two miles in, on an abandoned logging trail at the edge of a national forest. The victim's companion is to meet you and guide you in. The densely forested landscape is serene as you turn off the main road onto the poorly maintained logging trail. It is severely rutted and will probably be passable only to four-wheel drive vehicles after another winter has passed.

A lone female hiker frantically waves you down and tells you that her boyfriend is about 200 yards off the trail, where he was bitten by a rattlesnake (the only poisonous variety indigenous to this area). With drug kit and resuscitator in hand, you proceed after her on foot. Your partner follows with splints and a stretcher.

Once at the scene, you find a male patient in his early 20s. He is sitting on the ground; a tourniquet improvised from a belt is in place just below his left knee. Upon examination you find two puncture marks on the midcalf area. There is redness and swelling, about 10 to 20 cm in diameter, and the patient complains of extreme pain. You also note marked cyanosis below the level of the tourniquet. Checking for a distal pulse, you find none on the affected leg. You place a constricting band just above the tourniquet and then slowly release the belt until a weak pulse is palpable. Questioning the patient, you find that the bite occurred about 45 minutes prior to your arrival.

Incising the wound to remove venom

1. is performed by making crisscross incisions directly over the bite
2. is always recommended when more than one hour from a medical facility
3. is ineffective after 20 to 30 minutes from time of envenomation
4. should never be done in the field

Incising a rattlesnake bite is rarely indicated in a field setting. If done within the first three to five minutes after envenomation, up to 50 percent of the venom may be removed. It is, however, ineffective after 20 to 30 minutes. Of utmost importance is first determining if the victim has received any venom because 20 to 25 percent of all rattlesnake bites are not accompanied by envenomation. If the decision is made to incise the wound, it should be done lengthwise through each fang mark, 4 to 6 ml in length, and extending as deep as the penetration of the fangs. Suction should be applied continuously for 30 to 60 minutes.

Because over 30 minutes have elapsed since your patient was bitten, you will not incise and suction the wound. A check of vital signs shows that pulse is 110, respirations are 20, and blood pressure 118/90. The patient's skin is pale and slightly clammy. He also complains of numbness and tingling around his mouth and in his hands.

Rattlesnake venom may produce all of the following signs within the first few hours *except*

1. localized swelling, redness, or ecchymosis
2. muscle twitching and paralysis
3. hemolysis and coagulation defects
4. generalized weakness and nausea

The effects of all pit viper venoms are due to both enzymatic and nonenzymatic components. Together these can produce neurotoxic and cardiotoxic, as well as hemotoxic, changes. Because the toxin is an antigen, it may also produce signs and symptoms consistent with an allergic reaction, even anaphylaxis. While hemolysis of red blood cells and a decrease of the clotting factor (platelets) does occur, it is generally not observed until 36 to 48 hours after envenomation.

Your partner splints the hiker's lower extremity to prevent any unnecessary movement of the affected part. According to the patient, the snake escaped into a nearby rock outcropping after the attack. He is positive, however, that it was a rattlesnake because he heard it buzz just before he was bitten. He tells you that the reptile was about four feet long and had a characteristically triangular-shaped head. Together you and your partner place the patient on a stretcher and carry him to your rescue squad. You proceed out to the main road, where he is transferred to a waiting ambulance.

Once inside the ambulance, an IV is started with normal saline at a keep-open rate. The patient complains of nausea and increasing pain around the area of the snakebite.

Narcotic analgesia (i.e., morphine) for this patient

1. is not recommended
2. would be ineffective
3. should be administered IM
4. is the drug of choice

Morphine is not recommended for prehospital treatment of a snakebite victim. While pain experienced by the victim may be severe, MS will produce vasodilation, which may enhance circulation of the venom. In addition, morphine is a respiratory depressant that may have a potentiated effect when used with some snake toxins.

En route to the hospital, you notify the emergency department by radio that your estimated time of arrival is 15 to 20 minutes. Vital signs continue to remain unchanged, and the patient's overall status is the same. This patient will obviously require antitoxin and close hospital monitoring.

Once at the emergency department, the physician on duty examines the patient and orders a series of stat lab tests. In addition, the physician measures the circumference of the patient's leg above and below the bite in order to check serially the increasing edema. A skin test is done to determine if there is any allergic reaction to the horse serum base of the antivenin. It is negative, and the antivenin is given by IV drip.

Discussion

Poisonous snakes of various varieties are found in many areas of the United States. Particularly endemic to the southwest are several species of rattlesnakes that account for 75 to 80 percent of all human deaths by snakebite each year.

Rattlesnake bites are most common from March to October when members of this species are out of hibernation. Signs and symptoms are variable; however, the most reliable signs are pain, redness, and swelling around the puncture wounds. A victim may receive little or no venom, though fang marks may be present.

In the prehospital phase, treatment should proceed as follows. Calm the patient and prevent any unnecessary activity on his part. Apply a constricting band approximately four inches proximal to the wound to restrict only venous flow. Do not remove until after antivenin treatment has been started. Immobilize the affected part, again to reduce unnecessary movement. Give no analgesics, and never pack the limb in ice. Monitor vital signs carefully, and transport as soon as possible. Incise and suction the wound only if less than 30 minutes have elapsed since the bite.

Your patient recovers after receiving seven vials of antivenin. He is hospitalized for several days, however, to be observed for possible residual effects. A week after the incident, he returns to your station to offer his thanks.

CASE STUDY 10B: MRS. V. RODRIGUEZ

You are called to respond to an apartment complex for an unconscious female. While you drive, your partner checks a detailed mapbook to locate the address given. It is a large complex, and it is essential to park as closely as possible to the right apartment.

As you turn into the parking lot, a teenage girl frantically waves her arms overhead to summon you to the correct apartment. With your arms fully loaded with the drug box, cardiac monitor, radio, and resuscitator, your partner and you follow her to the front door, which is wide open. Inside you find a woman in her late 30s, lying on the living room floor. Her breathing is deep and rapid, her pulse is weak and thready, and she responds to your attempts to arouse her by moaning incoherently. Your partner, as patient medic, puts her on oxygen at 4 l, and then places the electrode pads for the monitor. You learn that the young girl is the patient's daughter. She is frightened but tells you that her mother is a diabetic. She found her in this condition when she came home from school. When you ask the girl about her mother's insulin, she tells you that it is in the refrigerator.

Insulin, a hormone normally secreted by the pancreas, is essential for metabolism because

1. it breaks down carbohydrates into usable sugars
2. it promotes transport of glucose into body cells
3. it stimulates the liver to release stored glucose
4. it combines with serum glucose to release energy

Although the precise mechanism is not fully understood, insulin promotes the active transport of glucose into the cells for metabolism. Without it, glucose remains in the bloodstream, and the cells begin converting fat and proteins into usable forms. The byproducts of this process lead to a metabolic acidosis.

In the refrigerator you find several vials of insulin labeled "U–100 N (NPH)" and "U-100 R (regular)." This is not surprising; diabetics normally mix two or more types of insulin for their daily injection. You ask the daughter if her mother took her insulin today. She replies that she does not know. Asked about any recent illnesses, she tells you that the patient has had the "flu" for the last three days. Your suspicions at this point lead you to believe that your patient is probably unconscious because of

1. alcohol intoxication
2. overdose
3. viral syndrome
4. diabetes

While any unconscious patient may potentially be an overdose, it is logical to assume from the history given that this patient's decreased level of consciousness is probably related to her diabetes. The differentiation between insulin shock (hypoglycemia) and diabetic ketoacidosis (hyperglycemia) can be a difficult one to make in the prehospital setting. In any event, the treatment is simplified since paramedics do not routinely administer insulin in the field.

Your partner gives you this additional information from the physical exam. Pulse is 100 and weak, respirations are 40 and deep, and blood pressure is 110/80. The patient has a buildup of dried secretions around her mouth and appears dehydrated. EKG shows a sinus rhythm.

You go to the radio to contact the hospital. After your initial radio report, the hospital orders a blood sample to be drawn for analysis, an IV to be started with normal saline, and 50 cc of 50 percent dextrose to be given IV. Which of the following would *not* be appropriate for this patient:

1. $D_{50}W$, 25 gm IV
2. draw preglucose blood sample
3. Glucola, 75 gm p.o.
4. normal saline to keep open

Glucola should never be administered to an unconscious patient because of problems of aspiration. A good rule of thumb with any medication given by mouth (Glucola, Ipecac, etc.) is that the patient should be able to hold the container and drink for herself. A patient too obtunded to do this is not able to protect her airway adequately.

Your partner advances the IV cannula, tapes it down, and carefully draws 6 cc of blood into a syringe for analysis. The IV line is then hooked up and run at 100 cc per hour. Next, your partner gives 50 cc of $D_{50}W$ IV push, and you prepare to transport the patient to the hospital. After two or three minutes, there has been no significant change in your patient's consciousness. Her respirations are still Kussmaul in nature, deep and rapid. This patient's respiratory pattern is significant because it represents

1. a compensatory attempt to reverse acidosis
2. the occurrence of irreversible damage to the brain stem
3. an indication that the condition is terminal
4. a cardinal sign of narcotic overdose

Kussmaul respirations, which are characteristically seen in patients with diabetic ketoacidosis, attempt to compensate for the metabolic acidosis by creating a respiratory alkalosis. Not only are body cells starved for glucose but they also are subjected to a low pH. Indeed, treatment will be aimed at decreasing serum glucose with insulin and increasing blood pH with sodium bicarbonate. In addition, other electrolytes will likely be out of balance and need adjustment as well.

En route to the emergency room you inform the hospital that there has been no improvement in your patient's status. She is still unconscious and inappropriately responding to verbal stimulus. It is reasonable to assume that she is unconscious because of her diabetes, but since she is not responding, you begin to consider other possibilities. Your treatment protocol for an unconscious patient would call for a narcotic antagonist such as naloxone (Narcan) to be administered. You decide to discuss this with the hospital. On the basis of your observations, you believe the Narcan is not indicated because

1. this patient has no known history of drug abuse
2. there was no evidence of narcotics at the scene
3. narcotic overdose produces respiratory depression
4. the patient exhibits classic signs of hyperglycemia

All narcotics and opium derivatives are strong CNS depressants with secondary respiratory depressant effects. A patient who is unconscious but maintains deep and rapid respirations is, therefore, very unlikely to have any significant amount of narcotic on board.

After a brief discussion, the hospital decides not to order Narcan. Within minutes you arrive at the emergency room. Your patient is taken inside, and an immediate glucose level is ordered on your blood sample drawn 10 minutes earlier. Not surprisingly, the lab test shows a glucose level of 346 mg percent. Normal serum glucose levels should be

1. 30–60 mg percent
2. 60–100 mg percent
3. 100–200 mg percent
4. 200–400 mg percent

A normally acceptable range for blood glucose is 60–100 mg percent. Outside this range, brain cells are especially affected. Too little glucose in the blood due to a relatively high amount of insulin robs brain cells of their only source of metabolic energy. In addition, these cells have a low tolerance for dramatic pH changes; thus, in both cases the patient's level of consciousness is impaired. Owing in part to the fact that hypoglycemia and hyperglycemia are often not clearly distinguishable in the field, treatment is aimed at the former, which is always a more acute condition. While additional glucose given IV or by mouth will not significantly worsen the condition of a patient in diabetic ketoacidosis, it can produce a dramatic and brain-saving effect in an insulin reaction.

Obviously this patient has an abnormally high glucose level and is admitted to the ICU in diabetic ketoacidosis.

CASE STUDY 10C: MR. W. BROCK

Your fire department is notified of a truck overturned on the interstate highway. For such an incident your normal response is two engines and a rescue unit. Nearing the accident scene, you encounter heavy traffic, and you note that two police vehicles have already arrived. Your rescue vehicle is stopped, and you pause briefly to survey the scene. Down a shallow embankment, off the shoulder of the highway, lies a large truck on its side. There is no fire and no sign of victims. The vehicle is badly damaged.

As you approach the truck you see the DOT (Department of Transportation) placard identifying the contents as radioactive material. Promptly you notify the officer in charge, who orders all rescue personnel to don full protection clothing. A firefighter from the engine company is designated to measure for possible radiation with a Geiger counter. The audible clicking of the device becomes a steady buzz as it nears the truck. You are given a dosimeter, which attaches to the outside of your clothing and will measure cumulative radiation to which you are exposed. At the front of the truck you peer through the windshield. You can see the driver still restrained by his seatbelt, suspended motionless in the cab. The rubber molding around the windshield is peeled away and the glass quickly pried out. Stepping inside the cab, you check for breathing and a carotid pulse. Both are present as your patient is apparently unconscious.

At this point you may assume that this patient's loss of consciousness is not due to

1. head injury
2. radiation exposure
3. cardiac arrhythmia
4. hypovolemia

Acute radiation sickness can produce malaise, fever, nausea, vomiting, and diarrhea within the first 24 to 48 hours, depending upon the whole body dose. Loss of consciousness acutely due to radiation exposure, however, is extremely unlikely; thus, other possible causes must be considered.

After placing a cervical collar on your patient, you release his seatbelt and, with the help of several firefighters, lower him gently onto a backboard. He begins to regain consciousness and complains of a headache, dizziness, and pain in his left shoulder. You decide to move the patient up the embankment, away from his vehicle, before examining him for further injuries.

Which of the following factors has the least influence on the amount of radiation your patient may have received:

1. strength and type of radiation
2. distance from the source of radioactivity
3. length of exposure
4. type of clothing worn

Since the type of radiation with which we are concerned most is so-called "penetrating" radiation (i.e., X-rays, gamma rays, etc.), clothing provides minimal protection. However, the cumulative dose, distance from the source, and duration of exposure influence how much damage may be expected from such radiation.

While you begin a complete physical exam of the patient, other rescue personnel cover the gurney, floor, and bench seat of the ambulance with plastic-backed disposable blankets. Although your patient himself is not radioactive, his clothing (as well as your own) contains radioactive particles that make them "contaminated." From the point of initial exposure, anything coming in contact with you, your patient, your clothing, or the immediate environment around the radioactive source will also be considered contaminated.

Your physical exam reveals a male patient in his late 20s. He is conscious but still somewhat confused and displays some short-term memory loss. His skin has normal color and is warm and dry. There is a small hematoma on the left temporal area; pupils are equal and reactive. Vital signs are pulse 96 and regular, blood pressure 132/86, and respirations 18. The patient complains of headache and dizziness; there is also pain and deformity near the distal end of his left clavicle. The rest of the neurological exam is normal, and his chest and abdomen are also negative. Having removed his clothes, you cover the patient with a sheet and splint his left shoulder with an arm sling. You also give him oxygen by nasal prongs.

Since you have controlled his present medical problems, your biggest problem is controlling contamination. The hospital has already been alerted to prepare for radiation isolation and decontamination procedures. Outside the ambulance window you can see that police have diverted the traffic flow, and fire department personnel have cordoned off a "hot zone" around the overturned truck.

En route to the hospital you review the physiological effects of irradiation. Which of these statements is not accurate:

1. severe radiation poisoning may lead to cardiovascular, GI, and CNS complications
2. radioactive particles remain in cells, causing tissue to become radioactive
3. radioactive particles on the skin can be washed off with soap and water
4. the onset of symptoms in radiation poisoning may not be seen until several days after exposure

Penetrating radiation passes through body tissues much like an electrical current. Damage may be done to cells, causing biochemical changes, but the tissue itself does not become radioactive. In addition, the onset of symptoms may be delayed from 24 hours to several days. Therefore, associated injuries should be treated first (i.e., fractures, bleeding, airway obstruction, etc.).

Upon arrival at the emergency room, you are directed to a little-used back entrance with your patient. Inside you are met by a team of doctors and nurses in full surgical scrubs, including shoe covers, masks, and gloves. All contaminated clothing is placed in a special bin for radioactive waste. You and your patient are bathed in an area designed so that wash water is recovered for disposal. Later, all other contaminated rescue workers must undergo similar decontamination procedures. The ambulance and other contaminated equipment are also out of service until decontaminated.

Discussion

The overall management of a radiation emergency is one of common sense. Once certain myths are destroyed and replaced with accurate information, procedures are very simple.

First, any patients should be treated the same as if they were not exposed. ABCs and standard treatment protocols should be followed. The patient is not radioactive, and rescue personnel need only protect themselves if possible from direct contact with contaminated clothing, etc. When practical, rescue workers should wear coveralls or surgical gowns, gloves, disposable masks, and shoe covers.

Protecting the environment and especially the ambulance and emergency room are also important as far as is practical. Covering the inside of the ambulance with paper, blankets, or sheets will make decontamination simple by disposal of any article that comes in contact with the patient (or rescue personnel if they are also exposed). The hospital should be notified as soon as possible so that steps can be taken there to deal with radiation decontamination.

Finally, remember the relative effects of dose, distance, and duration when faced with a radiation emergency. Terminating the patient's exposure to a source of radiation should always be the first step, with precautions to protect yourself if at all possible. Do not panic: A radiation emergency is no different from any other except perhaps in its mystique.

Your patient is found to have rather low levels of radiation poisoning. He also suffered a fractured clavicle. After observation for several days, he is discharged.

CASE STUDY 10D: MR. K. HENDERSON

"Squad 18 with Engine 7, respond to a possible drowning, 4262 La Grande Avenue, nearest cross street Springhill." You and your partner climb into your paramedic unit and simultaneously fasten your seatbelts. A brief two-minute response takes you to a public swimming pool in a local municipal recreation area. With resuscitator and monitor in hand, you precede your partner to a crowded poolside area where you find a lifeguard performing mouth-to-mouth resuscitation on a teenage male. While you set up the resuscitator to deliver 100 percent oxygen, your partner goes through the crowd with the radio and drug box. A check of the patient's respiratory status reveals that he is apneic; you ask the lifeguard to continue ventilating him, now with the valve and mask. His pulse is 50 and weak. With the monitor hooked up, you identify his rhythm as a sinus bradycardia.

This arrhythmia is most likely the result of

1. vagal stimulation
2. head injury
3. hypoxia and acidosis
4. alcohol intoxication

Sinus bradycardia is significant in this patient because it is probably the direct result of hypoxia and acidosis. In fact, primary field treatment is aimed solely at correcting these two acutely abnormal conditions. In drowning, as in cardiac arrest, when normal respirations cease, abrupt and immediate changes take place in arterial blood gases. Oxygen is quickly depleted and CO_2 rapidly builds up, producing a state both hypoxic and acidotic.

As patient medic, you begin an initial assessment of your patient. According to his companions, this 15-year-old boy was hyperventilating, then swimming as far as he could underwater. He failed to come to the surface, however, and was pulled from the water by the lifeguard. Upon examination you find that he is unconscious and unresponsive; both pupils are dilated and react sluggishly. His skin is pale, wet, and cool. When you auscultate his chest, you hear clear breath sounds during ventilation.

Clear breath sounds bilaterally confirm that

1. no aspiration has taken place
2. the patient is probably "faking it"

3. the patient has been in laryngospasm
4. none of the above

While breath sounds are important in evaluating the patient's ventilatory status, they confirm nothing at this point except that there is little or no fluid in the lower airways. Owing to its hypotonicity, fresh water is rapidly absorbed out of the lungs and into circulation. While "dry lung" due to laryngospasm is possible in this case, it cannot be determined strictly on the basis of clear lung sounds.

Your partner contacts the hospital by radio, describing the patient's condition and current critical status. By this time, with good ventilations being administered, his heart rate has increased to 68. The blood pressure is 108/60, and there are still no spontaneous respirations. The hospital orders an esophageal airway and an IV with D_5W to keep-open.

The use of an esophageal obturator airway in this patient

1. may be indicated, depending upon his size
2. should be via the nasopharyngeal route
3. will not prevent regurgitation of stomach contents
4. is unnecessary because ventilations are effective

The esophageal airway is used in the resuscitation of unconscious, nonbreathing patients provided that their size (not age) indicates its safe and accurate placement. While available models are unquestionably not for pediatric use, some teenage patients (especially male) may be successfully managed with this device.

Your patient appears to be large enough to accommodate safe placement of the EOA. After attaching the syringe and lubricating the obturator tip, you pass the airway with no difficulty. A recheck of breath sounds indicates proper placement, and you ask a firefighter from the engine company to continue ventilation.

Of the following drugs, which would you expect the hospital to order:

1. sodium bicarbonate, 1 mEq/kg IV
2. atropine, 1.0 mg IV
3. lidocaine, 1 mg/kg
4. dopamine, 200–400 mg IV drip

Although some controversy does exist, sodium bicarbonate is the only clearly indicated drug for this patient. Some physicians prefer to correct acidosis in the field strictly by means of hyperventilating the patient with 100 percent oxygen. This blows off carbon dioxide, thereby reducing the acidosis. However, depending upon the duration of immersion and the time elapsed before resuscitation, bicarbonate can and should be administered in most cases.

The hospital orders 70 mEq of sodium bicarbonate IV push for this 155-pound boy. The bicarbonate is given, and the patient is readied for transport. Ambulance personnel bring the gurney to the poolside area, and the patient is loaded onto it. A rolled-up towel under his shoulders helps to maintain a good, open airway. You hand the IV to one of the attendants and take over ventilating the patient as he is wheeled to the ambulance. Your partner follows quickly, with arms full of equipment.

Once in the ambulance you recheck vital signs. Blood pressure is 104/62; pulse is 70 and strong. There are still no spontaneous respirations, so you continue to ventilate at a rate of 24. The patient's overall status remains the same. Once you arrive at the emergency department, little time is wasted as the patient is transferred to the hospital gurney. The physician first checks lung sounds and pupillary response, then intubates the patient with an endotrachael tube. Blood gases, portable chest X-ray, a CBC, and electrolytes are immediately ordered and performed. With your job finished, you pick up equipment and supplies in order to return the squad to service.

Discussion

Prehospital management of a drowning (or if you prefer, neardrowning) patient differs little from treating a cardiac arrest. In fact, many times the patient may be both pulseless and apneic. In assuming that a palpable pulse is present, positive pressure ventilation with 100 percent oxygen to reverse hypoxia and acidosis is the most important treatment. Monitoring is essential, and arrhythmias are treated as needed. Associated injuries (i.e., cervical spine, head injury, etc.) should always be considered and treated accordingly.

Despite aggressive prehospital intervention, your patient develops severe pulmonary edema and dies two days later.

CASE STUDY 10E: MR. P. GROUSSARD

You are summoned to a private residence for a man with severe abdominal pain. Your response takes you into an elite area of expensive homes; you pull up a long winding driveway to a house overlooking a carefully manicured golf course. An attractive middle-aged woman meets you at the front door and leads you into the living room, where you find the patient lying on a sofa. As you introduce yourself and begin your physical exam, your partner questions the wife about any relevant medical history. Your patient is a male in his mid-40s with an acute onset of severe left upper quadrant pain. He is pale, warm, and dry. He complains of nausea and weakness and has been vomiting for two days. At first he ascribed his symptoms to be "just a touch of the flu," but he has been unable to keep anything down. Upon exam there are no masses; gentle palpation elicits pain in the left upper quadrant as well as voluntary stiffening of the abdominal muscles. There is a single surgical scar visible on the right lower quadrant, which the patient confirms as an appendectomy as a teenager.

The term that best describes this patient's abdomen is

1. rigid
2. rebound
3. guarding
4. flaccid

The abdomen is divided into four quadrants by imaginary vertical and horizontal lines intersecting at the umbilicus. When the belly is soft but there is voluntary contraction of abdominal wall muscles to palpation, the patient is guarding. A rigid abdomen is an involuntary response and may indicate blood in the abdomen or an inflammation of the abdominal lining (peritonitis). Rebound describes pain elicited by a rapid withdrawal of the examiner's hands during palpation.

The patient's vital signs are blood pressure 110/90, respiration 18, and pulse 150. Because his skin is warm to the touch, you also take an oral temperature, which is 98.8°F.

Having completed an initial primary assessment, you return to an investigation of the abdominal pain. Short, concise questions reveal the following information. He describes his pain as sharp and cramping at times. It does not radiate but is more severe when he tries to eat. When asked about his emesis, the patient tells you it is dark brown and very foul smelling. His medical history is unremarkable, and he takes no prescribed medications. He does suffer from occasional indigestion for which he takes Alka-Seltzer.

When you place electrode pads on the patient's chest and attach the chest leads, you see the rhythm shown in Figure 10–1.

This rhythm you identify as

1. junctional tachycardia
2. wandering atrial pacemaker
3. sinus arrhythmia
4. sinus tachycardia

Pain localized in the upper abdomen does not rule out a possible cardiac origin. An accurate history of the onset and quality of pain along with other factors, however, makes it unlikely that this pain is cardiac in nature. This patient's rhythm is in fact a sinus tachycardia with some artifact and is a normal response to the pain and apprehension.

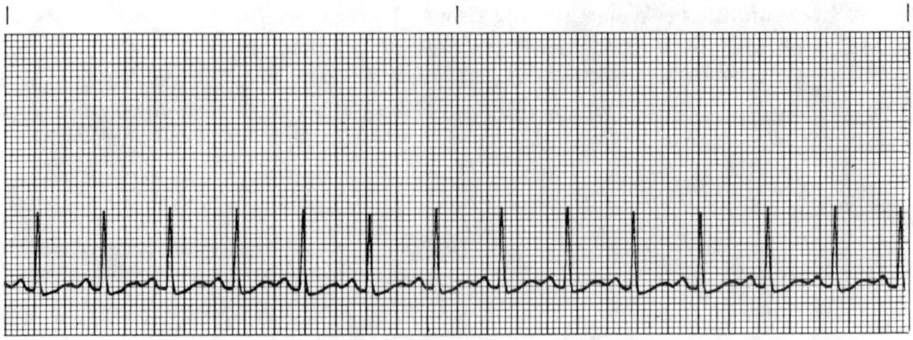

Figure 10–1. Rhythm Strip (Lead II)

Your partner contacts the hospital and sends an EKG strip. The physician orders an IV with normal saline at 200 cc/hr. After successfully cannulating a vein in the forearm, you tape the tubing securely in place. Your IV set is rated at 15 gtt/cc, and you adjust the drip rate to

1. 15 gtt/min
2. 200 gtt/min
3. 200 gtt/hr
4. 500 gtt/min

While not critical in this situation, calculations of IV drip rates in the field become extremely important when administering IV solutions containing medications. The proper drip rate for this patient can be calculated by multiplying the number of drops per cc (determined by the type of IV set being used) by the volume to be infused per hour and dividing by 60 minutes to obtain a drop rate per minute (see Table 10–1).

The patient is ready for transport. Though his pain status remains unchanged, you will not administer a narcotic analgesic, because his abdominal pain is yet undiagnosed. When you help him to stand up from his sitting position on the sofa, the patient begins to feel very weak and dizzy. The EKG monitor shows a slight increase in heart rate but no change in rhythm.

TABLE 10–1 Calculation of IV Drip Rate

$$\frac{15\text{gtt/cc} \times 200\text{ cc/hr}}{60\text{ min/hr}} = 50\text{ gtt/min}$$

Which of thc following procedures would you want to perform:

1. obtain orthostatic pulse and blood pressure
2. take bilateral blood pressures
3. increase the IV drip rate
4. pop an ammonia ampule beneath the patient's nose

Symptoms of weakness, dizziness, or syncope upon change of position from sitting to standing are most frequently attributed to vasovagal stimulation, arrhythmias, or hypovolemia. In such cases it will be helpful to obtain a blood pressure and pulse from both sitting and standing positions. A change of 20 beats per minute in heart rate or drop of 10 points in systolic blood pressure upon standing is indicative of hypovolemia.

A recheck of the patient's blood pressure shows a drop to 96/68 with an increase in pulse rate. The hospital is informed, and you are requested to run in 250 cc of IV solution as a fluid challenge. In addition, you place the patient on the gurney with his feet elevated on a pillow. Once in the ambulance a recheck of the blood pressure becomes more difficult because road noises randomly imitate the faint arterial sounds that you are trying to hear with the stethoscope. Upon arrival at the ER, however, his blood pressure is 120/80 after the infusion of 500 cc of IV solution. The patient is also able to sit up without feeling lightheaded. After examination by the emergency room doctor, the patient is given a panel of routine lab tests including urinalysis, CBC, amylase, enzymes, blood urea nitrogen (BUN), and creatinine. A full series of abdominal X-rays is also ordered.

Discussion

Diagnosis of abdominal disorders can be extremely difficult even for a physician in the hospital, where a final determination of the cause may only be possible by exploratory surgery. The prehospital treatment is basically supportive, but certain areas also should be routinely considered by the paramedic team. A good history and description of the pain, though only seldom diagnostic, are a logical starting point and may help rule out some disorders. Nausea and vomiting are a frequent chief complaint and should be explored as to onset, number of episodes, and description of the vomitus. The relationship of meals and beverages to the abdominal pain or vomiting may also be important. Changes in normal bowel habits should be asked (i.e., constipation, diarrhea, tarry or bloody stools, etc.). If the patient is female, there are also gynecologic considerations: last menstrual period, intermenstrual bleeding, possibility of pregnancy, etc.

Careful palpation of the abdomen should be carried out except in cases of a pulsating mass (indicative of a possible aneurysm). Auscultation of bowel sounds is rarely practiced in the field but when performed they should be reported as either present or absent. Owing to the possibility of hypovolemia from dehydration or hemorrhage, an IV line may be started with an isotonic solution as indicated. Of course, medical history should be explored for previous episodes of abdominal distress.

Finally a list of common abdominal disorders that may produce acute symptoms (Table 10–2) is certainly worth review. Test yourself as you recall the various pathophysiology involved with each disease or disorder.

Your 45-year-old patient is diagnosed as having bowel obstruction. He is scheduled for surgery and discharged one week later.

CASE STUDY 10F: MS. B. DOWNING

As you and your partner are returning to headquarters from a call, the fire department dispatcher instructs you to respond to a woman in a parked car with difficulty breathing. When you arrive at the scene you find a woman in her late 20s sitting behind the steering wheel of her car in the parking lot of a large shopping center. She is rather flushed and appears quite anxious. She tells you that her throat feels like it's closing up and she can't breathe. There is also urticaria developing on her back, chest, and abdomen. Her pulse is 140 and weakly palpable. Blood pressure is 90/60. Her breathing is rapid and shallow. Between breaths she is able to tell you only that she had been shopping and began to feel rather weak and lightheaded, so she returned to her car. A passerby, seeing her distress, promptly notified the fire department. Your partner auscultates diffuse bilateral wheezes on inspiration and expiration. You notify the hospital that you have a female patient in acute respiratory distress. You receive an order to start an IV line with lactated Ringer's. After receiving your physical assessment, the hospital requests that you give epinephrine 1:1,000 0.3 mg SQ immediately.

TABLE 10–2 Intraabdominal Disorders

Reflux esophagitis	Viral syndrome
Gastroenteritis	Appendicitis
Gastric ulcer	Bowel obstruction
Pancreatitis	Kidney stone
Pelvic inflammatory disease	Labor
Ectopic pregnancy	Spontaneous abortion
Herniated bowel	Malignancy
Cholecystitis	Urinary tract infection
Food poisoning	Abdominal aneurysm
Abdominal trauma	Peritonitis

How can you best measure the effectiveness of this drug:

1. heart rate increases
2. patient's anxiety is reduced
3. breath sounds improve
4. urticaria begins to disappear

When given for anaphylaxis, epinephrine has two primary pharmacological effects: It produces bronchodilation of the lower airways and peripheral vasoconstriction. These effects can be measured by serial auscultation of lung sounds and monitoring blood pressure. A decrease in the patient's level of anxiety, while desirable, is not an objective measure of the drug's effectiveness.

After moving the patient from her car and onto the gurney, she is put on high flow oxygen. The monitor is hooked up, and the IV is established with a large bore cannula. The epinephrine is injected subcutaneously into her left arm. A recheck of her vitals shows that pulse is 150, respirations are 36 and labored, blood pressure is 70/50. Lung sounds are unchanged. Your patient has become very agitated and confused. With the patient in the ambulance you advise the hospital of her deteriorating condition. They advise you to increase the IV drip rate to wide open. Five minutes after the initial dose, you are to give another injection of 0.3 mg epinephrine 1:1,000 SQ. The second injection is administered, but there is no change in the patient's acute status.

What is the most likely explanation for this patient's continued deterioration:

1. infiltrated IV
2. irreversible shock
3. acidosis
4. poor drug circulation

Frank anaphylaxis produces two life-threatening conditions: (1) severely compromised ventilation due to edema and spasm of the upper airway and bronchi and (2) relative hypovolemia due to peripheral vasodilation and pooling. Unlike other shock syndromes, where there is usually peripheral vasoconstriction, an anaphylactic reaction can respond to subcutaneous epinephrine because the peripheral vasculature is dilated. However, insufficient arterial pressure to circulate the drug results in continued patient deterioration.

After running in a liter of lactated Ringer's, there is still no increase in blood pressure. The hospital requests that you set up a dopamine drip, 400 mg in 250 cc D_5W. There is also another bag of Ringer's to hang, so you put the radio in continuous voice-transmit mode for "hands-free" communications. Your ETA to the hospital is six to eight minutes. The dopamine is piggybacked into the IV line and started at 20 microdrops per minute.

Which of the following side effects would most likely occur when administering dopamine to this patient:

1. hypertension
2. angina
3. ventricular irritability
4. increased heart rate

Dopamine is cathecholomine, which is useful in treating hypotension by increasing cardiac output and stroke volume without significant increase in heart rate. Angina is a rare side effect; if the dopamine is monitored properly, hypertension is unlikely. As with most cardiotonic drugs, however, dopamine can enhance ventricular irritability, especially in a hypoxic condition.

When you recheck the blood pressure, it is 84 systolic by palpation. Pulse is 140, and respirations are 28. It is most difficult to hear lung sounds because of road noise, but the wheezes seem to be diminished bilaterally. The EKG continues to show a sinus tach.

Upon arrival at the emergency room your patient's BP is 100/70. She is wheeled inside where the ED physician examines her and orders arterial blood gases, portable chest X-ray, and EKG. Benadryl is also given IV. As her condition begins to stabilize, the doctor congratulates you and your partner for your prompt and aggressive field treatment.

Discussion

The body's immunological response to invasion by a foreign protein (insect venom, various foods, drugs, etc.) is a complex series of reactions not yet fully understood. Localized reaction such as pain accompanied by redness and swelling can be quite uncomfortable but is not serious in itself. However, a systemic reaction with tightness in the chest, urticaria (hives), and warm flushed skin is indicative of anaphylaxis and may be life-threatening.

An anaphylactic reaction is not always easily recognized, especially in the field. Patients with allergies generally avoid all contact with known allergens. However, when anaphylaxis is suspected, these patients must be observed closely. Judicious removal of the patient's clothing and a thorough physical exam is mandatory. Cardiac monitor is essential, as are vital signs every three to five minutes, with strict attention to blood pressure. Epinephrine 1:1,000 subcutaneous is the drug of choice to reverse bronchospasm and vasodilatation. An IV with Ringer's lactate should be started as soon as possible to run at a keep-open rate unless hypotension is observed. Benadryl IV can be given following epinephrine to prevent further histamine reaction, but it will have little effect on the allergic reaction already in progress. If hypotension is present, fluid replacement should be initiated first. If the response to IV fluids is not adequate, dopamine—200–400 mg in D_5W—should be given until B/P is greater than 90 systolic. Airway management is critical, and oxygen should be given at a high flow rate as soon as possible. Severe respiratory embarrassment may necessitate assisting ventilations.

Your patient's severe allergic reaction is later attributed to some peanuts in a candy bar that she had eaten while shopping. She remains in intensive care for three days. She is later discharged in good condition.

CASE STUDY 10G: MISS A. LENARD

"Woman down, possible overdose." This is the third such call that you and your partner have responded to this shift. As you arrive at the residence, several police cars are already on the scene where a boisterous teenage party is in progress. You grab your gear and head into the house. Music blares from the living room as you pass down a hallway to a dimly lit back bedroom. On the floor you find a girl in her late teens who is conscious but extremely confused and disoriented. Her speech is slurred and difficult to understand. While your partner talks with some bystanders, you begin to examine the patient. Her skin is warm and dry and appears to be of normal color. Her pupils are both 6–7 mm but do not respond to penlight. There is no obvious sign of head injury. Her pulse is 126 and regular, respirations are 18, and blood pressure is 118/80. The monitor shows a sinus tachycardia. Your partner has found that the girl has been drinking, according to her friends, and that she may have taken some Elavil.

Elavil, a tricyclic antidepressant, is dangerous in an overdose because it may cause

1. severe hypertension
2. cardiac arrhythmias
3. urinary incontinence
4. increased intracranial pressure

When taken in sufficient amount, Elavil may produce a number of dangerous side effects. Particularly significant are EKG conduction abnormalities such as bundle branch block and AV blocks. In addition, Elavil will enhance the effects of alcohol and other CNS depressants.

A brief search of the bathroom by your partner turns up an empty prescription bottle labeled "Elavil 100 mg. Take one tablet daily." The date on the prescription indicates that it was recently filled, so the patient could have taken a dangerous dose. Your partner goes to the radio to contact the hospital. You are asked to establish an IV line and send a strip. Oxygen is also started.

Appropriate treatment of this patient may include all of the following *except*

1. syrup of Ipecac
2. EKG monitor
3. IV, to keep-open
4. physostigmine

Ipecac is contraindicated in symptomatic tricyclic poisonings, especially in the presence of an altered state of consciousness. In such cases further depressed levels of consciousness are predictable and may occur rapidly. Gastric lavage may be helpful and should be carried out with appropriate precautions.

As you start the IV, your patient is becoming less responsive. She is very lethargic and responds only minimally to verbal stimulus. The monitor continues to show a sinus tach, but the P-R interval indicates a first-degree block. These initial cardiac effects are of much concern to you since you realize that toxic blood levels are being reached. Prompt transport of this patient is indicated. With the IV established, she is loaded into the waiting ambulance. En route to the hospital the decision is made by the emergency physician to give physostigmine, 2 mg via IV Volutrol over two minutes.

The effectiveness of this anticholinergic antagonist is best measured by

1. increased heart rate
2. decreased heart rate
3. decreased secretions
4. pupillary changes

Physostigmine (Antiliuium) inhibits cholinesterase activity, thus producing a parasympathetic effect. This can be seen as a decrease in heart rate. In addition, increased secretions and an improved level of consciousness should also be observed. Depending upon the amount of tricyclic ingested, repeat dosages may be necessary.

After giving the physostigmine by volutrol over two minutes, you note that the patient's pulse is 94. Her level of consciousness, however, remains unchanged. She is quite lethargic and difficult to arouse. Intermittent suctioning is required to clear her airway of saliva. By turning the patient on her side, you find it easier to maintain the airway. Five minutes after the initial dose, an additional 2 mg of physostigmine is ordered. Again there is no change in the patient's mental status.

The lack of improvement in the patient's level of consciousness may result from

1. blood alcohol level
2. additional unknown substance ingested
3. hypoglycemia
4. all of the above

Any of the suggested choices could result in a continued decreased level of consciousness in this patient. Specific lab tests can rule out most of these in the hospital setting, but in the field what is obvious, may not be absolute. For example, drawing a blood sample and pushing IV dextrose, which was not done initially, may have been appropriate even though available history did not suggest it.

Once in the emergency department your patient is examined by the physician who orders an EKG, CBC, urinalysis, drug screen, and blood levels for alcohol and glucose. Results of the test show high toxic levels for Elavil and a high blood alcohol. After transfer to the intensive care unit, the patient is monitored closely, especially for cardiac arrhythmias.

Discussion

Overdoses involving tricyclic compounds are unfortunately common. The very nature of the condition for which these drugs are prescribed (i.e., depression) makes them a popular choice for abuse. Common sense usually dictates that they be dispensed in small quantities; nevertheless, toxic levels are reached with relative ease. Prehospital treatment is symptomatic, but the paramedic should bear in mind that these patients can deteriorate very quickly. Cardiac arrhythmias, congestive failure, seizures, and visual hallucinations are possible side effects of tricyclics and should be anticipated. Vomiting that is induced soon after ingestion is appropriate in an asymptomatic patient. Prompt transport and continuous cardiac monitoring are essential.

Your teenage patient has an uneventful recovery and is discharged two weeks after admission.

CASE STUDY 10H: MR. M. POLLARD

Your peaceful night's sleep is abruptly terminated as you are awakened by the phone ringing beside your bed. It is 3:30 A.M. On the other end of the line is the calm voice of the group leader of your volunteer search and rescue (SAR) team. The team is being mobilized to find a missing climbing party overdue in the rugged Three Sisters Wilderness Area of the Oregon Cascades. As an intermediate EMT and a member of the local fire department, you have been chosen because of your expertise in emergency medical care. Team members will rendezvous in one hour for the search area, about 45 minutes away. Despite the many drills in which you have participated, there is no way to avoid the feeling of anticipation as you quickly dress and step into the crisp predawn air.

Once you arrive at the search area, a base camp is established, and the team is briefed on the missing climbers. There are four members in the party, which was scaling a nearby peak and failed to return within a designated time. All are males in their late 20s with varying degrees of mountaineering experience.

By midafternoon the search has been fruitless. For two hours rain drenches the area, dampening both spirits and rescuers. Finally, with darkness beginning to close in and temperatures dropping rapidly, the climbers are found. Initial radio reports from the scene indicate that one of the climbers has been killed in a fall, another has suffered a broken leg, and the remaining two appear exhausted and cold. Medical equipment and supplies are sent from the base camp as soon as it is determined that the climbers cannot be brought down safely before nightfall. You are at the scene shortly and put in charge of medical treatment. Other members of the SAR team have erected bivouac shelters.

Before you evaluate the three patients, your primary concern with regard to possible hypothermia is to

1. administer small amounts of alcohol by mouth
2. obtain oral temperatures on each patient
3. terminate their exposure to the environment
4. determine wind chill factor

As with heat injuries, the first step in combating effects of hypothermia is to terminate the patient's exposure to the environment. Shelter, dry clothing, and heat should be used to accomplish this task. Alcohol, while generally producing a pleasant feeling of internal warmth for both the patient and rescuers, is not recommended because it produces vasodilation and increased heat loss.

After the three climbers are placed in a shelter, they are given dry clothing and are examined by you and another EMT. The first patient is a 28-year-old male with pain and swelling of his right ankle. There is a palpable distal pulse on the dorsal surface of his foot. A splint is applied to immobilize the joint. He has no other apparent injuries, and his vital signs are stable. The second patient is also a 28-year-old male who landed on his ice axe when the lead member of the climbing party fell. He has some tenderness and ecchymosis in his left upper abdomen. His pulse is 110, respirations are 20, and blood pressure 126/80. Patient 3 is a 30-year-old male. His only apparent injury is frostbite on the fingers of his right hand. He is still shivering but his vital signs are within normal limits.

At this point which patient presents the *greatest* potential for deterioration due to shock:

1. patient with ankle injury
2. patient with abdominal injury
3. patient with hand injury
4. the same potential exists for all

The patient with abdominal trauma has the most potential to develop hypovolemic shock. In addition, hypothermia is already placing increased demands on the body to maintain core temperature. As the body's compensatory efforts to maintain tissue perfusion come into play, hypothermia may become profound. Not only will an increased respiratory rate cause greater core cooling, but a cold IV solution at ambient temperature infusing to combat hypovolemia may directly contribute to a lower body temperature.

All three patients appear to exhibit symptoms consistent with mild to moderate hypothermia. Even with dry clothing and shelter, each continues to shiver and show signs of exhaustion. You estimate outside temperatures in the low 40s; a 10-mile-per-hour wind flutters the sides of the tent. A space heater is set up, and one of the team members heats chicken broth for the patients on a portable stove.

You continue to be most concerned about the patient with abdominal tenderness. He is shivering uncontrollably, and his verbal responses to your questions are slow and somewhat vague. A recheck of his abdomen shows increasing tenderness and guarding. His pulse is 120, respirations are 24, and B/P is 110/70. You decide that a warmed intravenous solution may be indicated for this patient. In addition you elect not to give anything to him by mouth, at least for the time being.

What is the best reason for withholding warmed fluids by mouth in this patient:

1. fluids by mouth do not significantly add to circulating volume
2. increased activity of the GI tract shunts blood from vital organs
3. rapid rewarming with hot liquids is undesirable in this patient
4. he will probably be a candidate for surgery

Prehospital care must be considered as only the first phase of definitive patient care. In-hospital procedures, though seemingly unrelated to the field, are actually a continuum of treatment already begun. Learning to recognize a patient in the field who may end up in the operating room and treating accordingly (i.e., giving the patient nothing by mouth, starting an IV with a large-bore cannula, etc.) can help avoid unnecessary delays.

The patient with the ankle injury and the other with frostbite are given warm fluids to drink. Since you have standing orders for IVs in your rural EMS program, you elect to start an IV on the third patient with Ringer's lactate, which you have carefully warmed inside your jacket with your own body heat. After infusing a liter of warmed IV solution, your patient begins to improve, and his vital signs become stable. The pulse is 80, respirations are 16, and blood pressure is 124/72.

By 6:30 A.M. the injured climbers have been evacuated by helicopter to a treatment center 40 miles away. Your job is done.

Discussion

Treatment of hypothermia is based on the immediate termination of the patient's exposure to a cooling environment and rewarming as soon as possible. Experiments by the U.S. Coast Guard in 1975 showed that inhalation of warmed, humidified oxygen was one rewarming procedure that might be utilized in the prehospital setting without potential side effects. "Paradoxical cooling" is one such side effect observed in peripheral rewarming techniques. As external rewarming is applied, vasodilation occurs in the periphery, which in turn circulates cooled blood back to the body core.

When the core temperature falls to 92° to 96°F, internal organs do not function properly, and mental judgment is impaired. Shivering becomes more intense, and lack of control in the hands, arms, and legs is apparent. At internal temperatures of 86° to 91°F, shivering becomes violent and uncontrollable, speech is slow and slurred, and the victim appears exhausted and drowsy. Between 80° and 85°F a victim of hypothermia will become unconscious, and death will follow rapidly. Because normal heart pacemaker autoregulation ceases at about 80°F, death due to hypothermia is normally the result of cardiac arrest.

Emphasis in the field should be placed upon providing dry clothing or blankets and a warm environment. Warm fluids by mouth are recommended for patients with mild to moderate hypothermia, depending upon associated injuries and level of consciousness. Associated injuries are treated normally, keeping in mind that shock may be enhanced in an exposure patient, and cold IV solutions should be avoided. Cardiac monitoring is also recommended to detect arrhythmias.

Your patient with the ankle injury has a fractured distal tibia and is placed in a cast for six weeks. The patient with left upper quadrant tenderness goes to surgery for a ruptured spleen. The patient with the frostbite injury is treated and released.

CASE STUDY 10I: MR. S. HOROWITZ

Like many paramedics with several years' seniority, you had requested and been approved a transfer to a "beach" situation for the next six months. Business is always brisk during the summer months when thousands flock to the ocean. During the past 30 days your unit has rolled on more than 200 calls.

The sun has hardly warmed the sand between the boardwalk and the water when you and your partner return to the station from your second call since 8:00 A.M., an overdose. Just as you sit down to finish the ever-present paperwork, the two-tone station alarm sounds off.

"Squad 16, respond to the U.S. Coast Guard station to assist on a helicopter rescue: diving accident. 4392 Harbor Boulevard. 0943 hours."

Pulling up to the main gate of the Coast Guard station, you shut down the red lights and siren. The guard gives you simple directions to the helicopter hangar apron where the HH3 helicopter is waiting. You both proceed to grab the necessary equipment from the squad. A helmeted member of the crew helps you into the helicopter and points to where you are to stow your equipment and hands each of you an orange life vest and communications headset and closes the hatch. In moments the helicopter lifts off and banks sharply to the left as it climbs out.

You are told by a crew member that a distress message was received by radio 10 minutes ago and that a scuba diver is in trouble. The diver is in or near a small fishing boat about six miles off the point and that you'll be there in three to four minutes.

Within a few minutes the helicopter is hovering 30 feet above a small inboard vessel rocking back and forth on the swells below. Two figures, both in wetsuits, can be seen in the back of the boat. One is motioning frantically to the helicopter.

"We'll send one of you down in this to check him out," shouts the crew member pointing to what looks like an overgrown birdcage resting on the helicopter's metal deck. "Take this portable radio and let us know what you need." Dry mouthed, you climb into the basket and swing out into the downdraft of the rotor wash to be lowered to the boat.

Once on the boat you proceed to the patient. The patient is a male in his early 20s and is obviously dyspneic.

"I think he's having a heart attack or something," his diving buddy says. "We'd been down about 20 minutes when we had to come back up because my regulator was fouled up. When we got to the surface he said his chest hurt and he couldn't breathe."

"Was he holding his breath on the way up?" you ask as you get out a stethoscope.

"I don't know, but this is his first ocean dive."

Which injury may occur if the diver does not exhale as he ascends:

1. nitrogen narcosis
2. air embolism
3. the bends (decompression sickness)
4. ruptured eardrum

The most common problem encountered by scuba divers on ascent is air embolism. As compressed gases in the lungs expand with decreasing pressure while ascending, the diver must exhale in order to equalize the pressure. If the diver does not, overexpansion of the air may cause the lung to rupture, producing a spontaneous pneumothorax.

Your patient is pale and short of breath. He is conscious, alert, and complains of severe right-sided chest pain. His vital signs are pulse 120, strong and regular, respirations 28 and labored, blood pressure 136/90. You put him on oxygen by mask and remove his wetsuit top. His lung sounds seem to be clear, but, with the helicopter hovering overhead, auscultation is nearly impossible. Upon palpation you feel crepitus on the anterior chest and neck which feels like "Rice Krispies" in a cellophane bag.

This crepitus is more correctly known as

1. hemoptysis
2. dead air space
3. mediastinal shift
4. subcutaneous emphysema

The presence of air trapped in the subcutaneous tissue is called subcutaneous emphysema. It can result from diffusion of gases through the pleura into the mediastinum and/or neck. It may have an edematous appearance and a crackling feel or texture.

By radio you signal the helicopter to lower the basket in order to transfer the patient off the boat. You believe his symptoms to be consistent with an air embolism. You quickly explain to the patient your intentions as the basket is maneuvered into position. He is then hoisted skyward and disappears through the open door on the starboard side of the helicopter. Moments later the basket reappears, and you are lifted aboard.

Once on board, the patient is hooked up to the cardiac monitor, which shows a sinus tachycardia. Vital signs remain unchanged.

The helicopter is now en route to the U.S. Navy Hyperbaric Test facility about 15 miles up the coast, where the patient can be subjected to recompression if necessary. In addition, the pilot intentionally flies at low altitude to reduce the possibility of further barotrauma to the patient.

Since positioning may be very important for this patient you should place the patient

1. head down in a left lateral position
2. supine with head elevated
3. prone with head turned to the side
4. in any position that is comfortable

A cerebral air embolism is probably the most hazardous complication that can accompany air embolism. The patient should be kept in a head down position (Trendleburg) to impede travel of an air bubble to the brain.

As you place several folded blankets beneath the foot of the Stokes litter, your partner contacts the hospital by radio. Although reception is poor because of the helicopter's low flight level over the water, you are approved to start an intravenous line to keep open. Oxygen is continued at 8 l by mask, and vital signs are monitored frequently. Blood pressures are palpated because of aircraft noise.

As the helicopter sets down at the Navy test facility, you are met by a physician and two assistants who are specialists in barotrauma. The patient is transferred to the recompression chamber for treatment.

Discussion

Air embolism is not the only significant injury or hazard associated with scuba diving. On the surface a diver may become entangled in kelp, buoy lines, etc. This may cause fatigue, panic, and could lead to drowning. Cold water can produce impaired judgment as well as other signs of hypothermia.

While descending, the diver may encounter difficulty in equalizing the pressure between the nasopharynx and the ears. Since the pain is generally self-limiting, failure to "clear" will usually result in a return to the surface rather than damage to the eardrum, sinuses, or middle ear.

At depth the diver can experience nitrogen narcosis, where dissolved nitrogen from the air breathed can affect cerebral function. This intoxicating effect is both depth and time dependent and may cause the diver to become careless about safety.

Finally, a diver may experience another injury if ascending from depths below 40 feet too rapidly: decompression sickness (or the bends). Nitrogen dissolved in the blood may not be absorbed quickly enough during ascent, causing gas bubbles to form that may block small blood vessels, creating a variety of signs and symptoms. Among these are pain in the joints, generalized fatigue, dizziness, visual disturbances, shortness of breath, convulsions, paralysis, or loss of consciousness. In severe cases the diver has to be treated in a hyperbaric chamber: The diver is taken to a simulated depth in order to redissolve the bubbles and then is brought back up gradually during several hours.

Your patient is treated at the hyperbaric facility and later transferred to a local hospital where he makes a full recovery.

CASE STUDY 10J: MR. M. JILES

The alarm clock on the nightstand dutifully awakens you at the pre-set hour of 6:00 A.M. This late-summer morning dawns much like each morning has in the last week, clear and hot. After dressing and fixing a light breakfast you drive to the fire station for your 24-hour shift. The digital sign in front of the local bank flashes the current temperature; it is already 85°. Fire hazard in the wildland areas of your fire district is extreme this time of the year, and the slightest spark is all that is necessary for several acres to be consumed by flames. Your station responds to brush fires nearly every afternoon, and today is likely to be no exception. Pulling into the parking lot at the fire station you note that hot winds are already whipping the flags nearly straight out from their mast. You estimate they are blowing 15 to 20 miles per hour.

The morning passes quietly as the emergency vehicles are checked carefully for proper levels of fuel, oil, and tire pressure. Equipment is cleaned and serviced as a part of a regular maintenance program.

By 1:00 P.M. temperatures outside are nearing 100° when the alarm comes in. "Station 34 respond to a wildfire, structures reported threatened, at Mountain View Road and Wild Oak Drive. Map 18, Delta 5."

You and your partner and the paramedic squad rush to the scene, the engine company following. Up ahead a large column of thick, brown smoke billows skyward. Already your flame-resistive safety clothing is causing you to sweat profusely. The squad and engine company are quickly assigned to protect homes from the fire, which has darkened the sky overhead with heavy smoke. Moving from house to house along the block your crew fights back the flames and the searing heat. The hit-and-run strategy seems to be working, and, with the help of a change in wind direction, the fire moves away from the homes.

As you and your partner are packing hose back into the fire engine, suddenly you begin to feel lightheaded and very dizzy. You feel yourself falling backward, and then everything goes dark. Within moments you are aware of your partner's voice calling your name. As you become aware of your surroundings, you find that you are lying on the ground, your feet elevated on a folded turnout coat.

"You must have taken a little too much heat and smoke back there," your partner says. "How are you feeling now?"

"A little weak I guess. What happened?"

"You passed out standing on the back of the truck."

Syncope is *least* likely to result from

1. cardiac arrhythmia
2. drug overdose
3. venous pooling
4. hypotension

Syncope is defined as a "transient loss of consciousness due to inadequate blood flow to the brain" *(Taber's Cyclopedic Medical Dictionary.* 13th edition). While drug overdose can produce a loss of consciousness, it is generally not transient in nature due to CNS effects, which may be prolonged.

Your partner grabs the drug box out of the squad and begins to check you out. How odd it feels, you think, to be the patient and not the paramedic. Your skin is slightly pale, warm, and very moist. You feel weak all over, and there are muscle cramps in both legs.

"Your BP is down a bit, 96 over 60," reports your partner. "Pulse is 120 and a little weak. I think you could use some IV Ringer's."

Thus far, your symptoms are most consistent with

1. transient ischemic attack
2. undiagnosed hypoglycemia
3. heat stroke
4. heat exhaustion

Given the preceding situation the most likely diagnosis lies between heat stroke and heat exhaustion. While heat stroke is the more severe condition, it does not usually present with the symptoms given. Instead, the patient will characteristically have dry, hot, and possibly flushed skin. Body temperature will also be high (104° to 108°F), and the patient may be disoriented, confused, or comatose. Pulse is rapid and bounding, and blood pressure may be normal or hypertensive. Rapid treatment is essential. In this case, heat exhaustion is the appropriate choice.

As the other firefighters help you out of your protective clothing, your partner sets up an IV. One of the crew gives you some oxygen by mask, and an ambulance is requested to respond to the scene. The intravenous line is started in a large vein in your forearm and taped in place. You are starting to feel somewhat better; however, the muscle cramps on your legs and now your arms continue to persist.

Heat cramps are directly related to

1. vasodilation in the periphery
2. loss of sodium due to sweating
3. overexertion causing muscle fatigue
4. lack of adequate circulation to muscles

Heat cramps may develop with excessive sweating, which also results in a loss of salt. When sodium levels fall below normal (hyponatremia), skeletal muscle function is impaired at the cellular level producing transient tetany or cramps.

With 500 ml of lactated Ringer's infused, your partner rechecks your vital signs. Your pulse is 90 and blood pressure is now 118/80. The ambulance has arrived at the scene to take you to the hospital to be checked out.

Your condition has improved significantly, and you ask to have your head elevated on the gurney. Your temperature is slightly above normal at 100.1°F when taken orally. Though you still feel weak, the muscle cramps are almost completely gone and you are somewhat embarrassed to be taken in by ambulance.

The most important reason for clinical evaluation of a patient following heat exhaustion is

1. detecting possible electrolyte imbalances
2. ensuring adequate rest and recuperation
3. monitoring the patient for cardiac arrhythmias
4. preventing the delayed onset of seizures

Heat exhaustion results primarily from loss of fluids and electrolytes, along with generalized vasodilation. While fluids can be replaced orally (in mild cases) or intravenously, electrolytes may also need to be corrected. Of course, an accurate determination of these values can only be carried out in the clinical setting.

Once at the emergency room you are given a warm reception by the ED staff. Your temperature and vital signs are taken, and blood samples are drawn for laboratory analysis. Following infusion of 1000 ml of lactated Ringer's solution, electrolytes have returned to normal limits, and you are discharged home for recuperation.

Discussion

Constant body temperature is maintained in a warm external environment in several ways. Increased temperature opens the skin pores and stimulates the sweat glands to increase perspiration. As perspiration evaporates, it cools the body. Increased temperatures also inhibit sympathetic tone, causing dilation of the peripheral vasculature which results in loss of heat through radiation. This produces some venous pooling, which can lead to a relative hypovolemia and/or hypotension. Finally, heat loss can be accomplished by evaporative cooling in the lungs through increased respirations. Under normal conditions, these cooling mechanisms function very efficiently and body temperature is regulated effectively. When the body's ability to maintain a homeothermic balance fails, the result may be either heat exhaustion or heat stroke.

Heat exhaustion. Heat exhaustion is brought on by loss of water and salt through sweating from exercise in a warm environment. Hypovolemia and shock develop as well as so-called *heat cramps* because of fluid loss, vasodilation, and hyponatremia. Signs and symptoms include wet and pale skin, weak and rapid pulse, hypotension, nausea and vomiting, muscle cramping, and syncope. Treatment should include cooling, fluids by mouth (if a mild case) or intravenously, and monitoring vital signs. Oxygen should be given at moderate to high flow rates.

Heat stroke. Heat stroke results from the failure of the body's normal cooling mechanisms, especially evaporative cooling by sweating. It is a true medical emergency. Patients with heat stroke exhibit hot dry skin and a very high temperature. In addition, it is not unusual to see mental confusion, seizures, or coma. The pulse is strong and rapid, and the blood pressure can be normal or high. Aggressive cooling treatment is mandatory and must be started as soon as possible. The most effective method is to immerse the patient in a cool bath, and an IV with lactated Ringer's is recommended. ECG should be monitored, because arrhythmias can occur, and oxygen should be given preferably by mask to increase concentrations. Vital signs should also be monitored closely, including temperature.

After resting at home for a day and a half, you are able to report for duty for your next shift. Being the patient for once, however, gives you some unanticipated insights into the special needs of the people who you take care of every shift.

RELATED ASSESSMENT QUESTIONS

10.1 For an unconscious patient, your first consideration should be to
- **(a)** look for identification
- **(b)** get a medical history
- **(c)** assess the airway
- **(d)** feel for a pulse
- **(e)** pursue the chief complaint

10.2 Signs of organophosphate poisoning include all of the following *except*
- **(a)** constricted pupils
- **(b)** diaphoresis
- **(c)** bradycardia
- **(d)** seizures
- **(e)** dry mouth

10.3 The usual dosage of Benadryl is
- **(a)** 25–50 mg
- **(b)** 50–100 mg
- **(c)** 100–200 mg
- **(d)** 250–500 mg
- **(e)** none of the above

10.4 Which of the following is *not* a side effect of physostigmine:
- **(a)** salivation
- **(b)** seizures

(c) urinary incontinence
(d) loss of bowel sounds
(e) bradycardia

10.5 The two primary concerns in treating a near-drowning victim are management of
(a) circulatory collapse and cardiac arrhythmias
(b) hypoxia and acidosis
(c) venous pooling and pulmonary edema
(d) peripheral edema and low cardiac output
(e) aspiration and depressed brain function

10.6 Victims of marine animal injury should be evaluated carefully because they might develop
(a) allergic reaction
(b) hypertension
(c) bradycardia
(d) thrombophlebitis
(e) pulmonary embolus

10.7 When a patient is known to have ingested a toxic quantity of drugs but is still awake and alert, the treatment of choice is
(a) Valium
(b) Ipecac
(c) Narcan
(d) dextrose
(e) physostigmine

10.8 Management of an unconscious patient who is suspected of drug overdose should probably include all of the following *except*
(a) IV
(b) EOA
(c) oxygen
(d) EKG
(e) Narcan

10.9 Which of the following is *not* included in the field treatment of heat stroke:
(a) change of environment
(b) large glasses of cold fluids orally
(c) ice packs to major artery sites
(d) Valium as needed to control seizures
(e) IV RL or NS to replace lost volume

10.10 Which of the following is *most* likely to be included in the treatment of acute, nontraumatic abdominal pain:
(a) IV and prompt transport
(b) sips of warm water

(c) hot packs to the abdomen
(d) N/G tube and MS for pain
(e) Ipecac and prompt transport

10.11 Before inserting a nasogastric tube, you should determine the appropriate insertion length by measuring
(a) twice the length of the patient's forearm
(b) from forehead to umbilicus
(c) from eye to clavicle to waist
(d) twice the distance from clavicle to xiphoid
(e) from nose to ear to xiphoid

10.12 Your patient, a female, has overdosed on tricyclic antidepressants. She is cowering in the corner of the room and hysterically asking you to put out the fire that she thinks is surrounding her. After assessing her vital signs and EKG, you will most likely be ordered to
(a) give atropine 2 mg IV push
(b) give Ipecac 30 ml orally
(c) give physostigmine 2 mg IV Volutrol
(d) give Narcan 0.4 mg IV push
(e) put out the fire and bring her in

10.13 The pain from a jellyfish sting can be reduced by
(a) giving morphine sulfate IM
(b) giving high flow oxygen
(c) immersing the limb in salt water
(d) applying meat tenderizer
(e) rinsing with alcohol

10.14 When administering 50 percent dextrose by direct IV push, you should watch closely for
(a) reflex bradycardia
(b) infiltration and subsequent necrosis
(c) peripheral vasodilatation
(d) ventricular irritability
(e) none of the above; this is a benign drug

10.15 Which of the following statements about an asymptomatic near-drowning victim is true:
(a) may require Valium to reduce anxieties
(b) should be given sodium bicarbonate prophylactically
(c) will be particularly prone to hypertension
(d) will likely suffer skeletal muscle seizures for 24 to 48 hours
(e) must be transported to the hospital for further evaluation

10.16 An N/G tube is used to
(a) suction the airway
(b) empty the bladder

(c) decompress the stomach
(d) occlude the stomach
(e) open the airway

10.17 The dosage of physostigmine is
(a) 5 mg in 500 ml 5 percent D/W, titrated to effect
(b) 25 mg deep IM
(c) 2 mg in 10 ml IV Volutrol over 2 minutes
(d) 10 mEq per kg body weight, repeatable once
(e) 0.5 mg IV push, repeatable in 20 minutes

10.18 Your patient is a 17-year-old boy who collapsed unconscious on the football field at school. His vital signs are normal, but his skin is cool and clammy. He is having slight skeletal muscle tremors. He has no ID on him, but he has what appear to be injection sites on his thighs. You would expect to give him
(a) Narcan IV
(b) Glucola PO
(c) physostigmine IV
(d) atropine IM
(e) 50 percent dextrose IV

10.19 Which of the following is the correct dosage for Ipecac:
(a) 30 ml
(b) 50 mg
(c) 75 cc
(d) 250 mEq
(e) 1 gm

10.20 Treatment of a snakebite victim includes
(a) encouraging ambulation
(b) elevating affected extremity
(c) soaking the injured limb in ice water
(d) applying a constricting band
(e) injecting epinephrine SC at the site

10.21 Indications that your patient is having a systemic allergic reaction include all of the following *except*
(a) hypertension
(b) rash and urticaria
(c) respiratory distress
(d) generalized edema
(e) laryngeal edema

10.22 Which of the following is the correct dosage for 50 percent dextrose:
(a) 50 gm IV push
(b) 500 mg IV push or orally
(c) 50 mEq IV push or IV drip

(d) 25 gm IV push
(e) 1 gm in 500 ml IV drip

10.23 Narcan is effective in reversing the effects of which of the following drugs:
(a) all injectable drugs
(b) all sedatives and narcotics
(c) only barbiturates
(d) only narcotics and opiate derivatives
(e) both barbiturates and analgesics

10.24 Which of the following would be most helpful in alleviating the pain of a stingray injury:
(a) give morphine IM
(b) immerse limb in saltwater
(c) rub sand on the wound
(d) apply heat
(e) pack in ice

10.25 The best thing that you can do for a patient with nonspecific abdominal pain is to
(a) give 2 mg MS IV
(b) insert an N/G tube
(c) auscultate bowel sounds
(d) palpate the abdomen by quadrants
(e) transport without undue delay

10.26 You respond to a home where a hysterical father tells you that he just pulled his baby unconscious from the bath tub. He says the child was left there a minute while he went to get a towel. The child is conscious and screaming. Your initial assessment reveals normal vital signs and clear lung sounds. You should
(a) transport the child to the hospital for further evaluation
(b) start an IV and give sodium bicarbonate
(c) give prophylactic Lidocaine in anticipation of arrhythmias
(d) give the baby high flow oxygen and draw blood gases
(e) hold the baby head down and suction to remove water from the lungs

10.27 The main systemic imbalances that present in both freshwater and saltwater drownings are
(a) pulmonary and cerebral edema
(b) hypoxia and acidosis
(c) atrial and ventricular fibrillation
(d) pulmonary edema and cerebral infarct
(e) cerebral edema and ventricular aneurysm

10.28 "Coffee-ground" emesis is an indication of
- **(a)** aspiration pneumonitis
- **(b)** septic infection
- **(c)** gall bladder trouble
- **(d)** GI bleeding
- **(e)** colitis

10.29 Which of the following would you use to treat a conscious diabetic who is symptomatic:
- **(a)** Glucola
- **(b)** insulin
- **(c)** sodium bicarbonate
- **(d)** 50 percent dextrose
- **(e)** orange juice with sugar added

10.30 Which of the following is a contraindication to the administration of Benadryl:
- **(a)** upper respiratory infection
- **(b)** alcohol intoxication
- **(c)** allergic reaction
- **(d)** hypertension
- **(e)** urticaria

10.31 Benadryl is used in the management of allergic reaction because it acts by
- **(a)** binding to histamine receptor sites to prevent further reaction
- **(b)** reversing existing reaction by toxifying allergins
- **(c)** preventing reaction by neutralizing histamine
- **(d)** alleviating symptoms by dilating bronchial tubes
- **(e)** releasing cathecholamines to overcome symptoms

10.32 Which of the following statements about syrup of Ipecac is *not* true:
- **(a)** it must be followed with water
- **(b)** it acts by stimulating the medulla and by irritating the stomach lining
- **(c)** the adult dosage is 30 ml
- **(d)** the patient's airway must be protected
- **(e)** it should not be given to children

10.33 Pharmocologic treatment of anaphylactic shock should include
- **(a)** atropine and Isuprel
- **(b)** dopamine and IV fluids
- **(c)** physostigmine and Aminophylline
- **(d)** Aramine and sodium bicarbonate
- **(e)** epinephrine and Benadryl

10.34 Which of the following is the correct dosage/route for Glucola:
- **(a)** 50 mg IV push
- **(b)** 250 mg IV Volutrol

(c) 30 ml orally
(d) 7 oz orally
(e) 25–50 mg IM

10.35 Prior to administering Glucola, you must
(a) check for presence of a gag reflex
(b) start an IV and give oxygen
(c) monitor the EKG for ventricular ectopics
(d) try Narcan to see if drugs are present
(e) insert an N/G tube

10.36 Which of the following statements about Narcan is *true*:
(a) it is ineffective against Darvon
(b) it can only be given by the IV route
(c) it has severe side effects if no narcotic is in the blood stream
(d) the initial dose is 5 mg
(e) it may need to be repeated as many as five to ten times

10.37 Which of the following is the most likely indication for the use of Benadryl:
(a) sedation prior to cardioversion
(b) asthma attacks
(c) allergic reaction
(d) suppression of ventricular ectopy
(e) hypotensive crisis

10.38 Prior to administering any form of glucose, you should
(a) draw a blood sample
(b) start an IV
(c) apply a cardiac monitor
(d) elevate the extremity
(e) dilute it with 20 ml sterile water

10.39 Treatment of organophosphate poisoning includes
(a) atropine and transport for further treatment
(b) Ipecac and referral for follow-up
(c) Narcan and prompt hospitalization
(d) atropine and Isuprel, then hospitalization
(e) thorough flush with weak vinegar solution, then release to a private physician

10.40 Which of the following can be used as diagnostic tools with a coma of unknown origin:
(a) epinephrine, EKG, and Benadryl
(b) glucola, mannitol, and EKG
(c) oxygen, Narcan, and dextrose
(d) Narcan and dopamine
(e) EKG and carotid sinus massage

10.41 You suspect that your patient has ingested an alkaline drain cleaner. Which of the following actions would be *most* appropriate:
(a) insert an EOA and monitor respiratory status
(b) give vinegar to neutralize the alkali
(c) give milk and transport immediately
(d) insert an N/G tube
(e) give Ipecac and watch the airway closely

10.42 Your initial concern in management of a patient in a coma is to
(a) determine the cause
(b) monitor the EKG
(c) elicit thorough history
(d) protect the airway
(e) start an IV and intubate

10.43 You are called to the local YWCA, where a young woman has fainted during gym class. Her skin is cool and moist, her blood pressure is 110/78, and her pulse is 92. She is now conscious and has a gag reflex, but she acts giddy and almost appears to be drunk. When questioned, she denies any current illness and says that her only past illness was sugar diabetes and the flu about two months ago. Your field treatment would most likely include
(a) ammonia ampule and oxygen
(b) oxygen and 50 percent D/W IV push
(c) a candy bar and IV fluids
(d) insulin and oxygen
(e) blood draw and Glucola

10.44. Epinephrine is useful in treating anaphylaxis because it
(a) binds with histamine to prevent further reaction
(b) prevents ventricular fibrillation
(c) constricts peripheral vasculature and relaxes bronchial tree
(d) dilates blood vessels and increases perfusion
(e) increases heart rate and decreases myocardial oxygen consumption

10.45 In an alert patient who has overdosed on Valium tablets, the most appropriate initial therapy would be
(a) oxygen by mask
(b) esophageal airway
(c) Narcan
(d) Ipecac
(e) physostigmine

10.46 In a patient who has been bitten by a poisonous snake, you can impede absorption of the venom by
(a) elevating the extremity and administering epinephrine
(b) lowering the extremity and applying a constricting band
(c) applying an arterial tourniquet and soaking in ice water

(d) administering epinephrine and having the patient walk
(e) applying rotating tourniquets and incising the wound

10.47 Your 42-year-old male patient has been vomiting brownish material for two days and is now vomiting frank blood. He is pale and has cold, clammy skin. His blood pressure is 82/60, pulse is 144, and respirations are 32 and shallow. Your management of this patient will include
(a) IV TKO, intubation, and gastric lavage
(b) nasogastric tube, IV RL, and rotating tourniquets
(c) volume IV fluids, antishock trousers, and prompt transport
(d) shock position, vasopressors, and antishock trousers
(e) sips of ice water, suctioning, and high flow oxygen

10.48 When atropine is given to treat organophosphate poisoning, the appropriate dosage is
(a) 0.5–1 mg IV push, titrated to effect
(b) 2 mg IV push, repeated as needed
(c) 5–10 mg IV push over 1 minute
(d) 15 mg slow IV push, repeated once if needed
(e) 20 mg deep IM

10.49 The initial dosage range for Narcan is
(a) 1–2 gm
(b) 250–500 mg
(c) 25–30 mg
(d) 5–10 mg
(e) 0.4–0.8 mg

10.50 Organophosphate poisoning should be suspected in any acutely ill
(a) aircraft mechanic
(b) asbestos worker
(c) cannery worker
(d) coffee taster
(e) farm worker

10.51 Your patient is a 9-year-old boy on a baseball field. He is conscious, dyspneic, and extremely anxious. His face is flushed and slightly swollen, and he complains of a throbbing headache and tightness in his chest. You should suspect
(a) asthma
(b) anaphylaxis
(c) migraine headache
(d) concussion
(e) epilepsy

10.52 Which of the following is *not* usually associated with systematic hypothermia
(a) difficulty in speaking
(b) flaccid muscle tone

(c) loss of memory
(d) decreased level of consciousness
(e) cardiac arrhythmias

ANSWER KEY

10.1 c	**10.14** b	**10.27** b	**10.40** c
10.2 e	**10.15** e	**10.28** d	**10.41** c
10.3 a	**10.16** c	**10.29** a	**10.42** d
10.4 d	**10.17** c	**10.30** b	**10.43** e
10.5 b	**10.18** e	**10.31** a	**10.44** c
10.6 a	**10.19** a	**10.32** e	**10.45** d
10.7 b	**10.20** d	**10.33** e	**10.46** b
10.8 b	**10.21** a	**10.34** d	**10.47** c
10.9 b	**10.22** d	**10.35** a	**10.48** b
10.10 a	**10.23** d	**10.36** e	**10.49** e
10.11 e	**10.24** d	**10.37** c	**10.50** e
10.12 c	**10.25** e	**10.38** a	**10.51** b
10.13 e	**10.26** a	**10.39** a	**10.52** b

11

OBSTETRIC/GYNECOLOGIC EMERGENCIES

CASE STUDY 11A: MRS. D. COLLINS

You are called to respond to a woman in labor. As the ambulance pulls into the street, you instinctively turn the heater switch full-on, providing a warm environment for the newborn.

Upon arriving at the residence you find a woman in her late 20s who is having strong uterine contractions every 2 minutes, each of which lasts 90 seconds. This is her third child, and she tells you that the baby is not due for another four weeks. Upon examination you observe fetal buttocks in the birth canal. A rapid decision is required: transport immediately or deliver the baby in the field. Of the following, what is the most significant information relevant to your decision:

1. strong uterine contractions two minutes apart
2. baby is crowning
3. mother is multipara
4. baby is premature

When the presenting part of the baby is visible at the floor of the perineum, delivery is imminent. Crowning is also accompanied by a strong urge to push as the baby applies pressure against the maternal rectum. At this stage the presenting part has already passed through the fully dilated cervix; under normal conditions, delivery of the infant is accomplished within a few minutes.

The decision is made to prepare for a breech delivery prior to transport. Your partner establishes communication with the hospital while you put the patient on high flow oxygen. As you glove up, the mother has another contraction, and her perineum bulges. At this point your primary concern is to

1. make a midline episiotomy
2. auscultate fetal heart tones
3. start an IV on the mother
4. prevent an explosive delivery

A rapid and uncontrolled delivery of the baby's head or buttocks presents a high risk of lacerating the mother's perineum. Subsequent hemorrhage could be profuse and difficult to control. In addition, bleeding represents an even greater hazard in controlling the airway of a breech baby, who normally will deliver face down.

The baby's buttocks and legs are gently and smoothly delivered. It is a girl. The infant is small as you would expect in a "premie," and you note that the lower extremities are cyanotic. You carefully help deliver each arm; the baby straddles your left arm, face down, with its head still engaged in the birth canal. This is the critical stage of breech birth. Your next step is

1. transport immediately, red lights and siren
2. deliver the baby's head by pulling on the torso
3. form an airway in the birth canal with your fingers
4. clamp and cut the umbilical cord

An adequate airway is always of first importance in any newborn. In a breech presentation, the cord may become compressed by the baby's head as it moves down the birth canal much the same as a prolapsed cord. With the baby's body already delivered, the infant may begin spontaneous respirations, which will require formation of an airway in the bottom of the birth canal. Without rapid intervention at this stage, the infant can quickly be asphyxiated. Also, there is a risk of damage to the cervical spine with the baby in this position; therefore, transport at this time can be extremely dangerous.

Within two minutes the baby's head is delivered. You continue to suction the airway, and you wrap the infant in a warm blanket. You note that the baby is cyanotic, particularly in the extremities, is rather listless, and does not cry readily. Pulse is 100, respirations are 40 and labored. You cut and clamp the umbilical cord. Your airway management should consist of repeated suctioning and

1. endotracheal intubation
2. assisting ventilations with bag and mask

3. oxygen at 4 to 6 l/min
4. mouth-to-mouth breathing

Oxygen should be used cautiously in newborns. Since damage to the immature retina can occur at relatively low flow rates using 100 percent oxygen, a good rule of thumb is to administer only enough oxygen to pink the baby up. The end of a connecting tube placed near the infant's nose can also be effective in providing an oxygen-enriched atmosphere. Repeated suctioning with a bulb syringe is imperative, with special attention to the nares. Premature infants are especially prone to periods of apnea because the lungs are one of the last organs to complete development in utero.

You have two patients on your hands. The mother appears to be doing well, and you ask your partner to take care of her. Your primary concern is the premature infant with some respiratory difficulty and a low initial Apgar score. You decide that immediate transport is indicated. The mother and baby are loaded into the ambulance to begin a 20-minute ride to the hospital.

As you continue to manage the airway and to stimulate her, the baby's condition improves, and she cries vigorously. Your ETA to the hospital is about seven minutes.

The mother begins to complain of abdominal pain, and the placenta delivers spontaneously. Suddenly there is a gush of blood, and your partner tells you that she is hemorrhaging profusely. You suspect that this bleeding is

1. normal, to be expected after delivery of the placenta
2. probably due to a laceration of the perineum
3. from the uterus, possibly a partially retained placenta
4. the result of a condition known as placenta previa

Although some bleeding is normal during the birth process, bleeding that is uncontrolled and profuse after delivery of the placenta is an ominous sign. Delivery of an incomplete placenta is a common cause of postpartum hemorrhage and may require intervention.

Your partner immediately begins to massage the fundus of the uterus as preparations are made to start an IV. Other appropriate field treatment to consider might be

1. Pitocin, 10–20 units IV drip
2. high flow oxygen
3. baby to the mother's breast
4. all of the above

Postpartum hemorrhage can rapidly result in hypovolemic shock for the mother. All of the above choices are appropriate. Rapid fluid replacement obviously should be kept in mind if these procedures are ineffective in correcting hypovolemia. In this case, Pitocin is used effectively to produce uterine muscle contraction, which controls the bleeding.

Upon admission to the hospital, mother and baby are taken to the obstetrical floor for follow-up care. Owing in part to competent and appropriate prehospital care, the mother is discharged in three days. Her now healthy baby daughter is released in three weeks after gaining weight in the neonatal intensive care unit.

CASE STUDY 11B: MRS. A. KNOTT

Your paramedic ambulance is dispatched to a ''woman down, possible beating, in a park.'' Your district is centered in an area of town with primarily low-income housing for minorities. Owing to the volatile nature of the neighborhood, you and your partner see victims of beatings, stabbings, and drug abuse on a regular basis. Not surprisingly, personnel turnover on your unit is the highest in the city, since burnout is common. Your partner grew up in a neighborhood of east Los Angeles not unlike this one. You work well together as a team; even the racial slurs hurled at you in the street are easily ignored.

''That park can get pretty rough at night,'' your partner says, as you jump into the ambulance cab. ''Check with dispatch to see if they are rolling a police cover unit with us.'' Automatically, you pick up the microphone and make the request.

''P.D. called this in, they're already on the scene,'' replies the dispatcher.

Police assistance should be requested for all incidents

1. where the commission of a crime is suspected
2. where a weapon is involved
3. where crowd control is necessary
4. all of the above

A request for police assistant is appropriate under many circumstances. However, response to your request may depend upon how well you have established a relationship with your law enforcement agency. Clearly, assistance should be requested (1) whenever you are prevented or restrained from carrying out your duty, (2) whenever you are suspicious that a serious crime is being or has been committed, and (3) whenever you are threatened with personal harm due to a person with a weapon. Other circumstances may include an uncooperative patient who refuses your help and yet requires further medical attention.

Pulling up to the scene you see two police cars parked with revolving red and blue lights, which reflect across the faces of 20 or more youths milling in the area.

One of the police officers approaches as you get out of the ambulance. "She was found about 10 minutes ago. She's pretty badly beaten, and we think that she may have been raped."

Huddled in the back seat of the police cruiser your patient is startled when you open the door. Crouching down beside the car you smile and introduce yourself as a paramedic. You can read the fear in her eyes as she draws away, saying nothing. Calmly you continue to speak, offering your willingness to help.

How would you deal with this patient:

1. request the police to question the victim regarding her assailant
2. use a gentle, empathetic approach; remove the patient to the privacy of the ambulance
3. be firm with the patient and complete the examination
4. wait for a female paramedic or police officer to assist you

A victim of sexual assault should be treated with gentleness and a nonjudgmental attitude. If possible, escort the patient to a place of privacy before beginning any examination. Provide a sheet or blanket to preserve modesty. Another female should be present during the examination for support and to avoid any later allegation of sexual misconduct on the part of the examiner.

With patience, you are able to convince the young woman to accompany you to the ambulance. A female police officer has also responded to the scene, and you ask her to join you. Switching off one set of overhead lights creates a less harsh environment inside the ambulance. You see that the patient is a woman in her early 20s. Her hair is disheveled, and there are multiple contusions on her face, neck, and forearms. There is also a small laceration in the corner of her mouth. Softly, you tell the patient that you would like to take her pulse and blood pressure as well as check her for other injuries. She nods her head and begins to cry, the first vocal response that you've had from her.

Which of the following is likely to present with a rape victim:

1. contusions, abrasions, or lacerations
2. bite marks
3. fractures
4. all of the above

Victims of sexual assault can sustain any of these injuries owing to physical trauma. While such injuries are usually found in areas of the genitals, buttocks, and breasts, other sites are also common. Treatment for these injuries is carried out in the usual manner.

The patient's vital signs are normal. A brief exam shows no other obvious injuries. She tells the policewoman her name but refuses to give any other information regarding the assault. En route you notify the hospital that your ETA is six minutes.

Once at the emergency department, your patient is accompanied by a nurse into a private examining room. Carefully, the nurse explains the details of the meticulous rape examination that the physician will perform with the patient's permission.

Discussion

Rape is a crime that leaves victims not only physically violated but stripped of dignity and self-esteem. Feelings of anger, humiliation, fear, blame, and even self-destruction are common. While the EMT or paramedic is rarely qualified as a professional psychologist, an understanding of these feelings and an empathetic attitude are important.

Owing to the violent nature of the victim's assault, traumatic injuries should be suspected. A history of the assault may be helpful but is not necessary. Examination of the genitalia need not be performed in the field unless obvious bleeding requires application of a dressing. Not only does this preserve the patient's modesty, but it may prevent unnecessary legal complications if the case is pursued in a court of law.

A victim of sexual assault can choose to refuse treatment. If the victim chooses to be taken to the hospital, encourage the victim *not* to wash, douche, or change clothing because these actions would affect collection of legal evidence.

Above all, treat a sexual assault victim with dignity and understanding. Exhibit a calm and professional manner, avoiding any sordid curiosity. Whenever possible, have another female present during examination and transport to the emergency department. Make certain that the ED staff recommends appropriate counseling for the patient.

Your patient is treated and released from the emergency room. She is referred to an active, nonprofit rape counseling agency for follow-up.

RELATED ASSESSMENT QUESTIONS

11.1 Management of postpartum hemorrhage includes all of the following *except*

(a) massage the fundus
(b) give IV fluids
(c) pack the vagina
(d) put the baby to breast
(e) give Pitocin

11.2 When Pitocin is given IM, the usual dosage is
- **(a)** 15–20 grains
- **(b)** 2.5–10 mg
- **(c)** 500 ml
- **(d)** 3–10 units
- **(e)** 5–15 mEq

11.3 During childbirth, a prolapsed umbilical cord should be treated by transporting promptly while
- **(a)** administering Pitocin
- **(b)** giving IV fluids
- **(c)** preventing pressure on the cord
- **(d)** applying the antishock trousers
- **(e)** monitoring maternal EKG

11.4 In addition to administering Pitocin to a patient experiencing postpartum hemorrhage, you should also implement which of the following measures:
- **(a)** IV volume expanders, antishock trousers, and EKG monitor
- **(b)** IV TKO, oxygen, and massaging the fundus
- **(c)** massaging fundus, IV fluids, and putting the baby to breast
- **(d)** IV fluids, packing the vagina, and placing in shock position
- **(e)** antishock trousers, shock position, and dopamine

11.5 Which of the following would not be an appropriate treatment for a rape victim:
- **(a)** assess and treat major trauma
- **(b)** cleanse the perineum with sterile saline
- **(c)** provide strong emotional support
- **(d)** allow a family member to be present
- **(e)** notify law enforcement agencies

11.6 Pitocin is used for control of
- **(a)** postpartum hemorrhage
- **(b)** tachyarrhythmias
- **(c)** blood pressure
- **(d)** bronchospasm
- **(e)** heart failure

11.7 Which of the following suggests that there is time to transport a primipara mother to the hospital before the baby comes:
- **(a)** the bag of water has broken
- **(b)** she has bloody show
- **(c)** crowning is only visible during contractions
- **(d)** the contractions are irregular, 45 minutes apart
- **(e)** she says that she has to have a bowel movement

11.8 Which of the following is not part of routine care for a newborn:
- **(a)** monitor respirations
- **(b)** clear the airway
- **(c)** monitor the EKG
- **(d)** maintain body temperature
- **(e)** determine Apgar score

11.9 What is your purpose in putting a newborn infant to the mother's breast immediately after delivery:
- **(a)** assures the mother that the baby is OK
- **(b)** stimulates the baby's respiratory effort
- **(c)** helps control postpartum hemorrhage
- **(d)** frees you to care for the mother
- **(e)** keeps the baby warm

11.10 During the delivery of an infant, you notice that the umbilical cord is prolapsed and presenting in the birth canal. You should
- **(a)** continue with the delivery as usual
- **(b)** quickly clamp the cord and then continue with the delivery
- **(c)** try to slip the cord over the infant's head and off the neck
- **(d)** use a gloved hand to prevent the baby's head from continuing down the birth canal
- **(e)** perform an episiotomy

11.11 Your initial assessment of a newborn girl reveals that she is active, crying well, and coughing. Her body is pink, her hands and feet are blue-tinged, and she has a heart rate of 120. You will assign her an Apgar score of
- **(a)** 12
- **(b)** 11
- **(c)** 10
- **(d)** 9
- **(e)** 8

11.12 Apgar scores are normally determined 1 minute after delivery and again at
- **(a)** 2 minutes
- **(b)** 5 minutes
- **(c)** 10 minutes
- **(d)** 30 minutes
- **(e)** 1 hour

11.13 In performing CPR on an infant, the proper technique calls for
- **(a)** two fingers over the middle of the sternum
- **(b)** a rate of 60 compressions per minute
- **(c)** a compression/ventilation ratio of 15:2
- **(d)** hyperextension of the neck
- **(e)** depression of the chest 1 to 1½ inches

11.14 A major concern in a patient with toxemia of pregnancy is
- **(a)** hypotension
- **(b)** fever
- **(c)** cardiac arrhythmias
- **(d)** cerebral hemorrhage
- **(e)** seizures

ANSWER KEY

11.1 c	**11.5** b	**11.9** c	**11.13** a
11.2 d	**11.6** a	**11.10** d	**11.14** e
11.3 c	**11.7** d	**11.11** d	
11.4 c	**11.8** c	**11.12** b	

12

PEDIATRIC EMERGENCIES

CASE STUDY 12A: TRACY E.

After delivering a patient to the emergency department, you sit down in the staff lounge with a glass of orange juice. Your partner puts your paramedic unit "available for response" over the portable radio and joins you. Before your partner can sit down, however, the radio comes to life. "Medic 3, respond to a child vomiting . . . 325 Hill Street." It looks like the start of another busy shift; this is your third call of the morning.

Pulling up to the residence your partner kills the master switch for the red lights and puts your unit "at scene" over the radio. You are met at the front door by a young woman in her 20s, holding a small child in her arms.

"It's my little girl, she's terribly sick," she says anxiously. "She started coughing and choking for no reason. Then, when she started vomiting, I called for the paramedics."

Gently, you take the child and carry her to the sofa in the living room. She is about two years old and cries softly as you examine her. Her skin is warm and dry. Pulse is 140 and regular as you listen to her chest with a stethoscope. Respirations are 48 and rapid; her breath sounds are clear. According to the mother, the child has not been ill recently and seemed normal only an hour earlier.

"Has the child been with you all morning?" your partner asks.

"Well, yes, of course. Except . . . when I was on the phone for about 20 minutes, and she was playing in the kitchen."

Quickly, your partner goes to check for possible clues. He soon returns with a nearly empty bottle of furniture polish in his hand. "This was on the floor by the sink. Do you remember how much may have been in the bottle?"

"I don't know, I'm not sure."

Which of the following is important with regard to poisoning:

1. identification of poison
2. amount of poison ingested
3. time since exposure
4. all of the above

All of the above parameters listed are important in poison emergencies and should be determined if possible. *Identification* of the poison is essential. When practical, obtain a sample or the container in which the product is found. The *amount* of poison ingested must often be estimated. In a 2- or 3-year-old, many researchers believe most ingestions are less than 30 cc (1 oz). *Time* since exposure may also have to be estimated in many cases.

A check of the patient's blood pressure shows 90/64. She continues to have an occasional nonproductive cough. You give her oxygen at 4 l by pediatric mask. Your partner contacts the hospital. After a brief discussion over whether to induce vomiting, you are requested to dilute the poison with water if possible. After an unsuccessful attempt to have your patient drink a glass of water, you prepare to transport the child.

Syrup of Ipecac is generally not indicated to induce vomiting of ingested hydrocarbons because

1. its use is contraindicated in children
2. there is high risk of pulmonary complications
3. hydrocarbons are too rapidly absorbed
4. hydrocarbons are harmless to the GI tract

Inducing emesis with ingested hydrocarbons (i.e., petroleum distillates) is controversial. Though emesis is advocated by some poison centers, there is a high risk with some hydrocarbons (e.g., gasoline, kerosene, lighter fluids, mineral seal oil) of pulmonary complications due to aspiration. These complications include pneumonia, pneumonitis, and pulmonary edema.

The hospital has contacted the poison center, and they do not recommend Ipecac for this patient. Therefore, you transport the young girl on her side in order to control any additional vomiting should it occur spontaneously. She has become increasingly lethargic.

At the emergency department, the patient is seen immediately by the ED physician, who orders a chest X-ray, arterial blood gases, CBC, urinalysis, and liver function tests.

Discussion

Poisonings constitute a significant emergency problem across the country. An estimated 10 percent of all emergency department visits can be attributed to drug overdoses, accidental ingestions by children, and other exposures to toxic substances. The prehospital care team is likely to encounter these patients frequently. Children are especially prone to accidental poisoning because ignorance and curiosity may lead them to sample the contents of a kitchen cupboard or bathroom medicine cabinet.

Poisons may be introduced into the body through a variety of routes: injection, absorption, ingestion, or inhalation. Acute hydrocarbon poisoning is most frequent by ingestion or inhalation. In the acute stage, from immediate postingestion up to several hours, symptoms may be seen as the poison affects the gastrointestinal tract. GI symptoms include nausea, vomiting, and abdominal pain. Only rarely is diarrhea an early symptom. CNS involvement is seen most frequently as depressed levels of consciousness ranging from lethargy to frank coma. Elevated body temperatures may also be present. Of greatest concern in hydrocarbon poisoning are effects on the respiratory tract. The hazard of aspiration during vomiting is obvious. In general, hydrocarbons are extremely toxic to bronchial tissues. Choking, coughing, and dyspnea are evidence that bronchial irritation is present. The patient may also exhibit stridor, tachypnea, and cyanosis with increasing respiratory distress. Pulmonary involvement is the most frequent complication from hydrocarbon ingestion.

Treatment is mainly supportive in cases of hydrocarbon poisoning. Airway management is of prime consideration, and high flow oxygen is indicated. Induced emesis may be recommended in some cases, as long as the patient exhibits an appropriate level of consciousness. Vomiting is often spontaneous due to GI irritation alone, and proper positioning to handle emesis should be encouraged. Dilution of the poison with water can and should be carried out in the prehospital phase. For severely poisoned patients, an intravenous line and continuous cardiac monitoring are recommended.

Your 2-year old patient is admitted for acute hydrocarbon ingestion and recovers after 10 days of hospitalization with specialized care.

CASES STUDY 12B: ANDY C.

Your paramedic ambulance is dispatched to a call for a child down. Your address takes you into a low-income housing area, and you consciously slow as children flock to the sidewalk to see your ambulance. As you turn down the street given, you search for street numbers. Age and carelessness have taken their toll because only an occasional house maintains a legible address. Finally the number is located, faded but visible, on an old mailbox, and you stop. As you approach the front door a woman's panic-stricken voice begs you to hurry. On the floor in the kitchen you find a young boy, his mother bent over him, frantically calling his name. While you go to the patient, your partner gently urges the woman out of the way. The patient is lying on his back and has generalized muscle twitching. He is about 6-years-old and is drooling large amounts of saliva from his mouth. He is unconscious and unresponsive.

Airway management is obviously of prime importance in this patient. Of the following, which would be an appropriate step in maintaining a patient airway:

1. oral suctioning
2. high flow oxygen
3. positioning the patient on his side
4. all of the above

While airway management is considered basic in proper patient care, it is occasionally performed inadequately in our rush to complete an assessment, identify an arrhythmia, start an IV, or administer medications. In this case all of the given steps are appropriate and desirable.

After turning the patient on his side and securing the airway, you continue to examine your pediatric patient. His pulse is 50 and weak. B/P is 90/60, and respirations are 16 and shallow. Pupils are constricted and equal. The EKG shows a sinus bradycardia. Meanwhile, your partner has obtained a sketchy history from the mother. The child has apparently been playing in the garage without supervision. He came inside the house, complaining of a stomachache and feeling very weak and dizzy. He then collapsed. The hospital is contacted via the paramedic radio, and EKG telemetry is transmitted. The hospital quickly orders an IV to be started with D_5W to run at a keep-open rate. Your partner also requests drawing a blood sample and the hospital agrees. While you look for a suitable vein, your partner sets up the IV, which includes a Metriset.

A Metriset (also called a Volutrol) is routinely used for pediatric patients because it

1. comes in several pediatric sizes
2. prevents inadvertent fluid overload
3. meters IV solution at exactly 15 gtt/cc
4. is easier to attach to a small bore IV cannula

Children have a relatively small intravascular volume, thus making fluid overload a significant problem in acute care cases. An in-line IV solution metering device allows accurate administration of small volumes and thus prevents inadvertent overload.

A blood sample is drawn, and the IV is started. The boy's pulse is 40.

Respirations and blood pressure remain unchanged. Intermittent suctioning is required to control oral secretions. The hospital requests the patient's body weight; you estimate 45 pounds. You are given an order to give 10 gm 50 percent dextrose slow IV. In the meantime your partner checks the garage for clues. The child's mother, though still very anxious, tells you that the boy has no medical problems. Your partner returns from the garage where an open container of insecticide was found. The label indicates that it contains the ingredient Parathion, an organophosphate (OP) compound.

Organophosphates enhance parasympathetic response of the automatic nervous system by

1. blocking acetylcholine receptor sites
2. suppressing sympathetic Beta receptors
3. binding to and deactivating cholinesterase
4. creating vagal nerve stimulation

Cholinesterase, an enzyme present at the synapse to break down acetylcholine, is inactivated by organophosphates. This results in uninhibited parasympathetic nerve transmission owing to excessive buildup of acetylcholine and produces cholinergic effects such as bradycardia, increased secretions, muscle weakness, and decreased level of consciousness.

Your partner quickly informs the hospital of the discovery. The hospital agrees that the patient's symptoms are consistent with acute organophosphate poisoning. You are ordered to give atropine 1.0 mg IV immediately.

Atropine blocks acetylcholine receptor sites at the synapse, thereby disrupting parasympathetic nerve transmission. Response to this drug can be measured by all of the following *except*

1. increased muscle tone
2. increased heart rate
3. decreased secretions
4. decreased cramping of the GI tract

While atropine indirectly produces a sympathetic effect (increased heart rate, decreased secretions, and decreased GI cramping), it has no effect on skeletal muscle tone. The therapeutic effect is best measured by monitoring the EKG and heart rate.

With 1.0 mg atropine on board, the patient's pulse increases to 50. No other significant changes are observed. The child remains unconscious; muscle tone is flaccid. You immediately load him in the ambulance and transport "red light and siren" to the hospital. En route, the hospital orders another 1.0 mg atropine IV.

Should you administer this additional dose of atropine?

1. yes, it has been ordered by the hospital
2. yes, multiple doses of atropine are often required in OP poisoning
3. no, there is already an observable effect in the increased heart rate
4. no, too much atropine can produce undesirable cardiotonic effects

Multiple doses of atropine are often necessary to reverse the cholingeric effects in OP poisoning. Even though this patient's pulse has increased, it is still in a bradycardia range and far less than a normal pediatric heart rate of 80 to 100.

In the emergency room your partner and you briefly discuss your patient's condition with the doctor. You assume that the child drank or was otherwise exposed to an unknown quantity of the insecticide, producing acute symptoms. More atropine is given to reverse the anticholinesterase effects. In addition, Protopam (pralidoxime) is administered to reverse skeletal muscle effects and reactive cholinesterase. Blood samples are drawn for specific lab tests, and the patient is transferred to the pediatric intensive care unit. He makes a full recovery and is discharged two weeks later.

Discussion

Pediatric emergencies most often seen by paramedics include poisoning, trauma, airway obstruction, and seizures. While treatment of children in general varies little from that of their adult counterparts, some important reminders should be mentioned.

Because children come in all shapes and sizes regardless of age, drug dosages are based on the child's body weight. For example, the correct pediatric dosage for atropine is 0.05 mg/kg. In our poisoned patient, this was calculated as follows:

$$0.05 \text{ mg/kg} \times 1.0 \text{ kg/2.2 lb} \times 45 \text{ lb} = 1.0 \text{ mg}$$

A conscious child who is injured or acutely ill is faced with an unknown and insecure environment when paramedics arrive. It is therefore important to get down to the child's eye level, talk calmly to the child, and reassure the child. In the case of an infant or toddler, try to let the mother or father hold the infant while you work.

Physiologically, a child has a larger surface area relative to body size than an adult. This can be especially important when treating patients with burns, exposure injuries, and absorption of toxic substances such as organophosphates.

Child abuse, unfortunately, is on the rise in this country. Child abuse crosses all socioeconomic boundaries. Whenever you encounter a child with suspicious injuries, an inconsistent history, or abnormal parent-child interaction, consider the possibility of child abuse. Be sure to relate suspicious facts to the physician who examines the child in the emergency room.

When it comes to prehospital care, children are not miniature adults. These patients require an intelligent and sensitive approach by the paramedic team.

RELATED ASSESSMENT QUESTIONS

12.1 In the absence of trauma, a stiff neck in a child is often an indication of
- **(a)** meningitis/encephalitis
- **(b)** airway obstruction
- **(c)** epilepsy/seizure disorder
- **(d)** pending sudden infant death syndrome (SIDS)
- **(e)** cerebral palsy

12.2 Which of the following statements is *least* correct regarding febrile convulsions:
- **(a)** they are caused by sudden temperature changes
- **(b)** they are usually self-limiting and require minimal treatment
- **(c)** initial treatment usually includes small doses of Valium
- **(d)** they usually respond to gentle cooling measures such as removing blankets and heavy clothing
- **(e)** these patients should always be transported to the hospital

12.3 In order to select an appropriate size pediatric endotracheal tube, you should choose one that
- **(a)** is the same size as the patient's age in months
- **(b)** is the same size as the patient's little finger
- **(c)** is as long as the distance from the nose to ear
- **(d)** fits snugly into the nares
- **(e)** is cuffed on the distal end

12.4 For a small child who has ingested an unknown quantity of aspirin but is conscious and alert, you should
- **(a)** insert a nasogastric tube
- **(b)** give Narcan
- **(c)** give milk
- **(d)** start an IV of Ringer's lactate
- **(e)** give syrup of Ipecac

12.5 Which of the following is specifically contraindicated in a pediatric patient suspected of having epiglottis:
- **(a)** IV fluids
- **(b)** external application of heat
- **(c)** Valium
- **(d)** high flow oxygen
- **(e)** visualizing the oropharynx

12.6 To defibrillate a child, you should use pediatric paddles. If for some reason these special paddles are not available, you should use the adult paddles. Which of the following positions best explains how you would modify your paddle placement to accommodate this improvisation:

(a) paddle 1: below right clavicle
paddle 2: at apex

(b) paddle 1: below right nipple
paddle 2: below left nipple

(c) paddle 1: anterior chest
paddle 2: posterior thorax

(d) paddle 1: immediately below midclavicular notch
paddle 2: immediately below xiphoid

(e) paddle 1: below left clavicle
paddle 2: at apex

12.7 You are ordered to defibrillate a 12-month-old male infant who appears to be of average build for his age. In order to determine an appropriate watt/second setting for this child, you will have to estimate his weight based on his age. Which of the following approximations would be the most accurate estimation of a 12-month-old's weight:

(a) 2 kg
(b) 10 kg
(c) 20 kg
(d) 30 kg
(e) 40 kg

12.8 An effective method of treating most asthma attacks in children is

(a) low flow oxygen
(b) IV Aminophylline
(c) breathing into a paper bag
(d) Benadryl inhalant
(e) epinephrine SC

12.9 A frequent complication of fever in a child is

(a) respiratory arrest
(b) hallucination
(c) loss of consciousness
(d) airway obstruction
(e) seizure

12.10 An asthma attack in a child is best treated with all of the following *except*

(a) a calm environment
(b) epinephrine SC
(c) high flow oxygen
(d) Aminophylline IV volutrol
(e) steam or humidified air

12.11 If your pediatric patient presents with fever, difficulty in swallowing, drooling, and inspiratory stridor, you should suspect that the patient might have epiglottitis and
- **(a)** give Aminophylline
- **(b)** intubate the trachea
- **(c)** avoid attempts at visualizing the larynx
- **(d)** insert an esophageal obturator airway
- **(e)** use Magill forceps and a laryngoscope to open the airway

12.12 Which of the following is the most appropriate treatment for a child with febrile convulsion:
- **(a)** immersion in ice water
- **(b)** alcohol sponge bath
- **(c)** IV fluids
- **(d)** gentle cooling measures
- **(e)** IV Valium

12.13 A 10-year-old child of average build will probably weigh
- **(a)** 40–50 lb
- **(b)** 60–75 lb
- **(c)** 80–90 lb
- **(d)** 95–110 lb
- **(e)** 110–125 lb

12.14 Which of the following is an essential component of a pediatric IV setup:
- **(a)** volume control chamber
- **(b)** extension tubing
- **(c)** in-line filter
- **(d)** multiple injection sites
- **(e)** plastic solution bag

12.15 Pediatric vital signs vary from those of adults in that pediatric
- **(a)** B/Ps and pulse rates are lower, but respirations are more rapid
- **(b)** pulse rates are slower, B/Ps are essentially the same, but respirations are more rapid
- **(c)** B/Ps are lower, but pulses and respirations are faster
- **(d)** B/Ps are higher, but pulses and respirations are slower
- **(e)** B/Ps and respiratory rates are higher, but pulses are slower

ANSWER KEY

12.1 a	**12.5** e	**12.9** e	**12.13** b
12.2 c	**12.6** c	**12.10** d	**12.14** a
12.3 b	**12.7** b	**12.11** c	**12.15** c
12.4 e	**12.8** e	**12.12** d	

13

MANAGEMENT OF THE EMOTIONALLY DISTURBED

CASE STUDY 13A: MR. F. COLDWELL

Your paramedic unit is dispatched to a local bowling alley for a person "acting strangely." It is normal policy for your paramedic agency simultaneously to request assistance from law enforcement personnel on such calls, but they are not yet at the scene when you arrive. It is about 8:00 P.M., and the parking lot is filled with cars when you reach the building. You and your partner are met at the front door by the manager of the bowling alley.

"He is one of our regular customers. I think he's sort of flipped out. All of a sudden he just started smashing up one of our scoring tables with his bowling ball . . . scared his wife half to death. He's always been a real nice guy, never caused any trouble."

With this information, what will you do first:

1. immediately attempt to restrain the patient
2. ask the manager to evacuate the building quietly
3. consult with the patient's wife for additional history
4. wait and do nothing until the police arrive

In this case, obtaining more information about the patient from his wife could be particularly helpful. Family members can frequently provide clues as to the nature of the disorder. While the other options could become necessary when dealing with such a patient, none are indicated at this time.

The manager shows you to his small office where he introduces you to the patient's wife. Meanwhile, three police officers have arrived and are standing by to assist as needed. From the office door you can see the woman's husband sitting behind the ball return ramp, his face buried in his hands.

"I've never seen him like this before," the wife says. "He has been under a lot of stress at work lately so we both thought that this would be a relaxing way to spend the evening."

Quickly you ascertain that the patient's name is Frank Coldwell and he is 46. He has been in generally good health and takes no medications. He seldom drinks and has never had any psychiatric disorders. He had two glasses of wine with dinner before coming to the bowling alley.

From this history you can safely rule out

1. undiagnosed hypoglycemia
2. alcohol intoxication
3. acute stress reaction
4. none of the above

It is extremely difficult to eliminate any probable causes of behavioral disorders in the field. Often the history may be suggestive; however, it is unwise to draw conclusions based solely on such information.

You and your partner approach the patient, who remains seated.

"Mr. Coldwell, my name is," and you give him your name and your partner's name. "We are paramedics. We're here to help you if we can."

"Did they send you here to get me?" your patient responds cryptically.

As you stand back, your partner approaches the patient and kneels beside him.

"We were called by the manager," your partner says. "He was concerned that you might hurt yourself or someone else."

"Then you must be one of them. They've been trying to get me."

It appears that your patient is not dealing in reality.

The best approach to take is to

1. go along with the patient's fantasy for the time being
2. let the patient's wife try to talk to him
3. allow the police to place him in custody
4. reinforce your identity and willingness to help

It can be extremely frustrating when trying to communicate with a patient of this kind. His disorder, regardless of the underlying cause, manifests itself in the present inability to deal in reality. A common sense approach in which we reinforce factual information such as our identity and willingness to help, though difficult, is recommended.

"Mr. Coldwell, we are paramedics and we're just here to help you," your partner repeats patiently. "Your wife has asked us to help you see a doctor."

The patient has exhibited no aggressive behavior since your arrival and in fact appears quite docile. Your partner is able to assess the man's vital signs. His pulse is 80, blood pressure 160/100, and respirations 16. His wife tells you that there has been no recent head injury. The patient agrees to accompany you to the paramedic unit; the wife is to follow you to the hospital.

While you contact the hospital your partner completes the exam, which is unremarkable. Suddenly the patient goes into a grand mal seizure. Your partner manages to place a bite stick between the patient's teeth, and you both struggle to protect him from hurting himself inside the confined space of the ambulance.

The seizure is clonic in nature and subsides after two minutes. Immediately you start oxygen by mask, but the patient remains unconscious. You inform the hospital of the change in the patient's condition. After less than a minute the patient has another seizure. The hospital requests that you start an IV with normal saline and give Valium, up to 10 mg to effect.

Which of the following is *not* true about Valium (Diazepam):

1. should be given rapidly to prevent precipitation
2. may cause respiratory depression or arrest
3. can produce a burning sensation on administration
4. has a cumulative effect with alcohol

While Valium does precipitate with some drugs and IV solutions, it should never be given rapidly. Rather, it is best administered slowly in 2.5 mg increments titrated to effect. Patients with behavioral disorders are rarely sedated in the field; thus, Valium is indicated in this case primarily for seizures.

Following the second seizure your partner is able to establish an IV line. Since the Valium is titrated to the seizure, your partner waits to give it until another begins. While seizures may occur with some psychiatric disorders, you and your partner suspect an organic medical problem.

Your patient remains unconscious as the Valium controls his seizure activity. You can transport him to the hospital. En route, your partner hooks up the cardiac monitor and continues to manage the airway.

Once at the emergency department the patient is transferred to a hospital gurney and the physician joins you. The initial exam shows the patient to be unconscious and unresponsive. Reflexes are normal, and vital signs are stable. Pupils are equal and reactive. The lab is called for blood tests; 50 percent dextrose is given without effect. A neurological consultation is requested, and the patient is sent for a CT scan, which reveals an intracerebral tumor.

Discussion

Patients with behavioral disorders are often difficult to manage. Since few paramedics are qualified psychologists, their role is primarily supportive. Our own aversion to the patient's actions or language may inhibit our effectiveness; it is important to keep personal emotions and value judgments in check.

Occasionally these patients can exhibit aggressive behavior and may perceive you as a threat to their safety or an ally of their enemies, real or imagined. Approach these patients cautiously and determine if a calm manner and quiet speech can be effective. If restraining patients for their own safety or that of others becomes necessary, do so humanely and quickly. Often more assistance may be required; check your resources first.

More often a calm nonthreatening approach can be used to gain their confidence, regardless of whether they are behaving aggressively or passively. Accurately reflecting their concerns as verbalized to you and expressing your desire to help frequently produce positive results.

Obviously, medical emergencies such as overdose, hypoglycemia, hypoxia, are treated normally. Patients who are depressed, emotionally disturbed, or exhibiting psychotic behavior may also have a very real organic problem that can easily be overlooked and might even be treatable in the field.

Quiet transport to an appropriate medical facility should be carried out in most cases, especially if the patient continues to display aberrant behavior after your arrival. Getting the patient into the ambulance may have a beneficial effect, because you can then control the environment. The use of red lights and siren can be disturbing for the patient; they should not be used unless a life-threatening emergency exists.

Your patient undergoes delicate surgery for removal of the tumor detected on the brain scan. After a period of rehabilitation, he exhibits no neurologic dysfunction.

RELATED ASSESSMENT QUESTIONS

13.1 Your patient is displaying bizarre behavior, which you suspect is some type of psychotic disorder. In addition to protecting yourself and the patient, you might also attempt to

(a) give oxygen and dextrose and transport promptly
(b) give oxygen and check deep tendon reflexes
(c) start an IV and monitor the EKG
(d) give IM Valium, restrain the patient, and transport "red lights and siren"
(e) check the pupils, give Narcan, and monitor closely

13.2 Your *primary* role in prehospital management of a behavioral disorder is to
(a) elicit a detailed mental history
(b) deliver the patient to the hospital without injurying anyone
(c) notify private psychiatrist
(d) counsel the patient against abuse of drugs/alcohol
(e) determine whether parents had a mental disorder

13.3 A person who exhibits signs of paranoia, delusions of grandeur, and schizophrenia should probably be under the care of a
(a) family physician
(b) psychiatrist
(c) marriage and family counselor
(d) neurologist
(e) neurosurgeon

13.4 Restraints should be used to protect
(a) the patient
(b) the paramedic
(c) other rescuers
(d) hospital staff
(e) all of the above

13.5 An overdose of which of the following drugs commonly produces dangerous and severe psychotic behavior:
(a) narcotics
(b) barbiturates
(c) Valium
(d) PCP
(e) phenothiazines

13.6 Your patient just found her 3-month-old infant asphyxiated in the crib. You determine that the baby has been down too long to be resuscitated. When you tell the mother, she becomes wildly hysterical. You might consider giving her
(a) Valium
(b) oxygen
(c) an ammonia ampule
(d) syrup of Ipecac
(e) an alcoholic beverage

13.7 Many emotionally disturbed patients respond best to
(a) clear, concise orders
(b) other family members
(c) a calm, empathetic approach
(d) oxygen therapy
(e) transport with "red lights and siren"

13.8 Which of the following causes of behavioral disorders can be effectively treated in the field:
(a) hallucinogen overdose
(b) alcohol intoxication
(c) severe depressive state
(d) brain tumor
(e) low blood glucose

13.9 Your patient claims that she has a green frog on her shoulder, even though you see nothing. You would describe this as
(a) a delusion
(b) a vision
(c) a hallucination
(d) a realistic fear
(e) a conversion reaction

13.10 The dosage of 50 percent D/W to rule out hypoglycemic behavior is
(a) 25 gm IV push
(b) 50 gm IV Volutrol
(c) 50 gm IV push
(d) 75 gm orally
(e) 80 gm IV Volutrol

13.11 You have been called by a woman who says that her husband is going to commit suicide. Upon arrival, your job will be to do all of the following *except*
(a) interview the patient to clarify the situation
(b) name the type of depression involved
(c) identify immediate threats to the safety of the patient or others
(d) relay information to the hospital so that the physician can direct disposition
(e) transport to an emergency psychiatric facility

13.12 Your female patient says that she has taken 50 Librium tablets because she wants to die. You are skeptical because you can't find any empty containers. You check her vital signs and EKG, and everything appears normal. You should
(a) leave your phone number with instructions to call if symptoms develop
(b) point out that she's abusing the system and leave
(c) refer her to the psychiatric outpatient department
(d) tell her to call her own physician
(e) give Ipecac and transport just in case

13.13 Which of the following is *not* a good approach to a behavioral emergency:
(a) express your concern and desire to help
(b) be calm and directive

(c) place yourself between the patient and the door
(d) approach the patient slowly and with sensitivity
(e) use the patient's own words to describe the problem

13.14 The most appropriate dosage when giving Valium to control acute stress reaction is
(a) 2.5 mg IM, titrated
(b) 5–10 mg IM
(c) 15–25 mg IM
(d) 50 mg IM
(e) 75–100 mg IM

ANSWER KEY

13.1 a	**13.5** d	**13.9** c	**13.12** e
13.2 b	**13.6** a	**13.10** a	**13.13** c
13.3 b	**13.7** c	**13.11** b	**13.14** b
13.4 e	**13.8** e		

14

RESCUE TECHNIQUES

CASE STUDY 14A: MR. T. STEVENS

At 5:00 P.M. routine daily activities around the firehouse are normally suspended. One or more members of the crew begin to prepare the evening meal; others may switch on the television. Such is the case at your headquarters station this evening. One of the top stories on TV is a "rescue in progress" of a climber with his leg caught in a rock crevice just north of your district. Live aerial footage from the TV station's news helicopter shows the hapless climber barely visible above a huge granite outcropping. The afternoon shadows growing long reveal the true ruggedness of the area's terrain. A full report is to follow on the news at eleven.

Nearly two hours later the station alarm sounds, and you are dispatched to the rescue scene. You are requested to bring in the fire department's Hurst "jaws of life" for the extrication attempt, which is 3½ hours old. The jaws of life is the most effective extrication tool to use for situations in which

1. the victim is located some distance away from the rescuers
2. glass must be broken to reach the victim
3. metal, wood, or rocks must be spread apart to release the victim
4. working space around the victim is very confined

The Hurst tool, or jaws of life, is used to spread objects, such as the rock crevice in which the climber's foot is caught. Its opposing jaws can be inserted into the crevice, where you hope that they will slowly spread until the crevice widens enough to remove the leg.

Twilight fades into darkness as you arrive at the staging area some two miles from the victim's location. A sheriff's department Hughes 500 helicopter is standing by in an adjacent field to ferry personnel and equipment to the site. After a quick briefing the engine company officer directs you to load the jaws aboard the helicopter and accompany it to the rescue scene. The officer will follow with additional equipment on the next trip.

The tool is loaded while you climb into the right seat of the helicopter, and the helicopter takes off. The pilot switches on the landing light, illuminating a 10-foot by 20-foot landing area on top of the chaparral-covered hilltop. Once on the hilltop you are amazed how rugged the area actually is, with huge granite rock formations and thick head-high sumac brush. You are told that the victim is around the other side of the summit and downhill some 200 feet from the landing area.

For 10 minutes you struggle to reach the site that you had seen earlier on TV. It feels odd to be there. Standing on top of a final rock formation you get your first glimpse of the victim and his two rescuers, one a paramedic and the other a reserve police officer who had been initially summoned to the scene by the victim's climbing companions. The 19-year-old victim is sitting astride a 10- to 12-inch-wide granite wall some 15 feet high. His right leg is lodged up to the groin in a 4- to 5-inch crack formed between the smaller granite piece on which he sits and the larger "parent" stone upon which you stand. Several attempts have been made to lift the victim out but it is impossible. Which of the following is probably contributing to the inability to free the climber's leg:

1. swelling
2. cold
3. shock
4. all of the above

Your continued efforts to free the leg will undoubtedly cause swelling, which serves to wedge the leg tighter into the crevice. On the other hand, both cold and, if present, shock, should work to your advantage.

Owing to the tremendous size of the rock, using the Hurst jaws to spread the crack is clearly beyond the capacity of the tool. It is nearly 8:00 P.M.

The victim, a local college student, had been rock climbing in the area with two companions, filming their activities for a class project. At 3:30 P.M. his footing slipped and his leg was jammed into the crack. Unable to free him, his companions hiked down to the lakeshore and summoned help from two police officers on patrol for poachers in the area. One of the patrolmen climbed to the location and, after surveying the situation, requested help from the county sheriff's department. In the meantime, several methods had been tried to free the young man's leg with no success. Cold soda, ice water, and motor oil were used in an effort to reduce soft tissue swelling and provide lubrication. Initial examination of the patient by paramedic personnel found him to be in some pain but otherwise in good spirits. His vital signs were stable. At 6:45 P.M. your fire department was requested to respond with the Hurst tool in the hope that the crack could be spread even a fraction and the victim's leg could be freed.

Soon the fire department captain shows up at your location and has brought 300 feet of kernmantle rope and two climbing harnesses. Even with flashlights turned off, the scene is bathed in soft moonlight. As the officer examines the situation, you find a spot to anchor the ropes that you will use as safety lines while working to free the victim. Cautiously you make your way down the steep slope of the massive rock to the outermost edge where the victim is trapped. The moisture of the evening air is making the rock face slippery, and the ropes are a necessity.

Slipping down beside the victim, your partner and you both tie off your ropes to prevent further descent. Looking down into the crack with a flashlight, you can see that his leg is pinned from just below the knee to his upper thigh. The crevice is nearly uniform in width both forward and behind his leg. His cut-off shorts allow the skin to abrade painfully against the stone. What might you do in order to minimize this complication:

1. slip gauze between his leg and the rock
2. give him something for pain
3. lubricate the leg
4. start an IV in case the bleeding worsens

After deciding that lubrication may be helpful, you select a large syringe from the paramedic drug box and fill it with motor oil. Then attaching it to a large-bore Teflon IV catheter, you inject the viscous fluid all around the leg. With some effort you are able to secure a nylon strap underneath the victim's foot like a stirrup in order to give him resistance to push against. With the captain standing behind the victim and lifting under his arms, you attempt to pull up on the strap. The victim cries out in pain and you are forced to abandon the idea. The night air is cooler and the victim, clad only in short-sleeves, complains of the cold. Slipping out of your turnout coat, you place it around his shoulders.

Finally it is determined that the only feasible solution is to chip away at the inside of the granite wall in an effort to create more space and relieve the binding pressure on the victim's leg. An air chisel with spare bottles is called for and flown to your location by the helicopter. In addition, you request a generator and floodlights. Fog is beginning to move in, causing concern about how much longer the helicopter can continue to fly. You glance at your watch by flashlight; it is 10:00 P.M. The sheriff's reserve search and rescue team is called in to aid in transferring the victim down the hill.

After explaining to the victim what you are about to do, you begin chiseling away at a small rock lip just behind his thigh. Occasionally a large chip is dislodged, but mostly it comes off as fine powder. The first air bottle is quickly drained and is replaced by another. The chisel tip, designed for cutting automobile sheet metal, is already dulled. Three more air bottles are emptied and your muscles begin to ache. The county fire department has sent another crew to relieve you. After applying liquid dishwashing soap to the victim's leg for additional lubrication, they continue to chisel at the rock wall. Looking around, you see 20 or more rescuers standing by to help wherever they can.

Finally, minutes before midnight, the chiseling stops. One last pull and the climber is free. His leg, though bruised and sore, appears okay. He is secured into the Stokes stretcher by the search and rescue team and carried uphill to the waiting helicopter, which flies him to the staging area. The rescue has taken eight and one-half hours. Equipment is carried to the landing area, where rescuers and their tools are systematically ferried down the hill.

The young man is transported to the emergency room, where he is treated and released with only minor contusions. News media covering the story report his gratitude to the countless persons who had a part in his rescue.

RELATED ASSESSMENT QUESTIONS

14.1 When treating a trauma patient with possible cervical injury, immobilization of the spine should be carried out immediately after assessing
- **(a)** pulse
- **(b)** airway
- **(c)** breathing
- **(d)** pupils
- **(e)** deep tendon reflexes

14.2 An automobile's front windshield glass is always made of
- **(a)** tempered glass
- **(b)** unbreakable glass
- **(c)** plate glass
- **(d)** safety glass
- **(e)** tinted glass

14.3 When gasoline is found leaking from a hole in the fuel tank, the best course of action is to
- **(a)** fill the tank with water to dilute the gasoline
- **(b)** make the hole larger to drain the tank quickly
- **(c)** flush all the gasoline into a storm drain

(d) remove any patients from the vehicle immediately
(e) plug the leak with a sealing compound

14.4 Tempered glass windows found in all vehicles are usually
(a) bulletproof
(b) easily broken
(c) located in side or rear windows
(d) harmless when broken
(e) used only for windshields

14.5 Which of the following is *least* safe for use as a personnel lifeline:
(a) manila
(b) polypropylene
(c) cotton
(d) kern-mantle
(e) all of the above are unsafe

14.6 Cribbing is utilized in vehicle rescue for
(a) protecting occupants from flying glass
(b) stabilizing the vehicle
(c) removing steel door posts
(d) cutting open the roof
(e) sliding the patient onto a backboard

14.7 Which of the following tools might be used to open a vehicle door jammed after a collision:
(a) pry bar
(b) hydraulic spreaders
(c) come-alongs
(d) halligan tool
(e) all of the above

14.8 Arriving at the scene of a vehicle accident, you find one of the autos in flames with a single occupant in that car. Your first priority when reaching that patient is to
(a) open the airway
(b) check the pulse
(c) remove him from the vehicle
(d) apply a cervical collar
(e) determine unconsciousness

14.9 Your patient is a butcher with a hand caught in a meat grinder, is in severe pain, and vital signs are stable. You should probably give
(a) Valium, slow IV
(b) epinephrine, SQ
(c) Benadryl, deep IM
(d) Dopamine, IV drip
(e) morphine, IV

14.10 When disconnecting a vehicle battery, it is best to
- **(a)** remove the positive terminal first
- **(b)** remove the negative terminal first
- **(c)** cut the positive cable with wire cutters
- **(d)** drain the electrolyte fluid first
- **(e)** remove the keys from the ignition first

14.11 A gasoline-powered rescue saw is rarely used for vehicle rescue because it
- **(a)** is noisy and may frighten the victims
- **(b)** cannot be used to cut metal
- **(c)** requires a minimum of two operators
- **(d)** causes too many sparks that may ignite the fuel
- **(e)** can be used on horizontal surfaces only

14.12 Which of the following is not used for immobilizing the spine:
- **(a)** backboard
- **(b)** cervical collar
- **(c)** antishock suit
- **(d)** sandbags
- **(e)** scoop stretcher

14.13 Which of the following is the best device to use when moving a nonambulatory patient over rugged terrain:
- **(a)** ambulance gurney
- **(b)** Stokes stretcher
- **(c)** surgical lift
- **(d)** wooden backboard
- **(e)** fireman's drag

14.14 A boating accident victim is pulled from the water mumbling incoherently and shivering uncontrollably. You should treat the victim for
- **(a)** hypothermia
- **(b)** hypotension
- **(c)** hypoglycemia
- **(d)** hypokalemia
- **(e)** hypochondria

14.15 Which of the following methods is *least* safe when rescuing a person stranded on top of his car in 3½ feet of fast running water:
- **(a)** toss a rope to the victim from shore
- **(b)** approach the victim with an inflatable boat
- **(c)** wait until the water level subsides
- **(d)** throw a life jacket to the victim
- **(e)** attempt a swimming rescue

ANSWER KEY

14.1 a	**14.5** a	**14.9** e	**14.13** b
14.2 d	**14.6** b	**14.10** b	**14.14** a
14.3 e	**14.7** e	**14.11** d	**14.15** e
14.4 c	**14.8** c	**14.12** c	

15

COMMUNICATIONS AND MULTIPLE CASUALTY INCIDENTS

CASE STUDY 15A: MR. R. WALKER

Your 24-hour shift starts with a routine check of your paramedic unit. Daily, the incoming paramedics assigned to your station are expected to go through the ambulance, making sure that drugs and supplies are stocked, as well as checking that telemetry equipment is operational. As radio medic for the day, you are also responsible for performing a radio check with a local hospital. As expected, the paramedic radio is functioning normally.

Shortly after 9:00 A.M. you are dispatched to a "man not breathing." Once at the scene you do in fact find a male victim approximately 165 lbs who is pulseless and apneic. Since your EMS program permits advanced airway management and an intravenous line to be established in such cases prior to any contact with the hospital, your partner selects an appropriate size endotracheal tube, while accompanying fire department personnel start CPR. Meanwhile, you start an IV line in the patient's right arm. The EKG monitor is hooked up and shows asystole. After gathering some pertinent information from bystanders, you make an initial radio report to the hospital. The physician immediately orders 1 mg epinephrine 1:10,000 IV and also requests EKG telemetry.

Which of these is not necessary in order to transmit EKG telemetry from the scene:

1. cardioscope
2. strip recorder

3. paramedic radio
4. radio-to-monitor cable

Most frequently, the EKG signal travels from the patient via a shielded cable to a portable cardiac monitor. From there it proceeds through an interconnect cable to the paramedic radio, where it is transformed into an audio signal. It is then transmitted to the hospital via radio or telephone. A strip recorder, though valuable in documenting rhythm strips at the scene, is not required to send EKG telemetry to the hospital.

The patient responds to initial treatment as you identify ventricular fibrillation on the monitor. Your partner quickly greases the paddles with conductive gel, charges the defibrillator, and delivers a countershock.

Any portable defibrillator should be capable of all of the following *except*

1. causing momentary contraction of the patient's skeletal muscles when current is delivered
2. allowing the operator to monitor cardiac rhythm when paddles are placed on the chest
3. producing a tingling sensation in the operator's hands as current is delivered
4. allowing selection of several different energy levels for defibrillation

All defibrillator units should provide complete protection to the operator from exposure to electrical shock when the unit is being properly used. Of course, any direct contact with the patient or a conductive surface during defibrillation will result in potentially hazardous electrical current being delivered to the rescuer.

The patient remains in V fib, but, after a second defibrillation, the rhythm converts to a slow sinus bradycardia with multifocal PVCs. The pulse rate increases to 48; CPR is stopped as pulses become palpable. Still in respiratory arrest, the patient requires ventilation with a positive pressure resuscitator.

Although recognizing that the heart rate is still slow, the hospital is very concerned that the ventricular ectopy may produce another episode of VF. You are asked to push Lidocaine, 75 mg IV. You feel, however, that atropine might be more appropriate to eliminate the PVCs.

The best course of action is to

1. give the Lidocaine as ordered without question
2. suggest that atropine be tried initially and followed with Lidocaine
3. transport the patient immediately since you can't agree
4. make an attempt to contact another hospital

The hospital considers your suggestion to try atropine first. However, not wishing to increase any potential infarct with an increased heart rate, the hospital elects to go ahead with a Lidocaine bolus. Since you can now understand the reasoning given, you administer the Lidocaine and make a mental note to discuss the issue with the physician.

Suddenly your patient begins to vomit; as your partner rolls him onto his side, you grab the suction catheter. The hospital is requesting an update on the patient's condition and also another rhythm strip.

Since both of you are tied up managing the airway, which of the following would be the best solution:

1. ignore the hospital's request for now
2. let your partner handle the airway himself
3. comply immediately with the hospital's request
4. place the radio in an "open transmit" mode and report information while assisting your partner

The hospital can only visualize what you tell them. When patient care requires two pairs of hands, the radio can be set to transmit voice communications continuously. This frees the radio medic to assist as needed.

Within minutes you arrive at the emergency department with your patient. Vital signs have stabilized, although the patient remains unconscious. The hospital staff continues treatment; a bed is readied in the coronary care unit.

As radio medic, you are responsible for completing the prehospital care form, which is utilized throughout your EMS program. The form includes all necessary patient information and treatment prior to arrival at the hospital.

Which of the following is *not* considered a necessary function of the prehospital care form:

1. to provide data for statistical evaluation
2. to provide a standard format for record keeping
3. to legally document treatment carried out by paramedics
4. to identify chronic abusers of the EMS system

This form or one like it is used by many EMS programs. While identifying system abusers is not a function of this record, the form is helpful in providing a standard format for record keeping as well as data for statistical evaluation. In most areas it is considered a legal document and may become a part of the patient's permanent hospital records.

You complete the paperwork while your partner places clean linen on the gurney and restocks supplies. As you are preparing to return to your station, the emergency physician asks you to join him in the doctor's lounge for some coffee. He informs you that your patient has suffered an inferior myocardial infarction and is in the CCU, doing well. He congratulates you both on the excellent job that you performed in the field.

CASE STUDY 15B: MULTIPLE CASUALTY INCIDENT

You and your partner have just settled in with a bowl of popcorn to watch a video movie you've rented. It's 9:00 P.M. on a Friday night, and no sooner have the credits rolled when multiple tones go off over the loudspeaker. The call is for a bleacher collapse at a local high school gymnasium with multiple victims. Your medic unit will probably be first in. You've participated in numerous disaster drills in the last five years but have never had to actually do it for real. Tonight could be a genuine test of your skills and ability to manage perhaps scores of real victims with not just plastic wounds and theatrical blood.

As your unit pulls up in front of the school gym located near the parking lot, you are immediately besieged by a crowd of pleading teenagers. The doors of the ambulance are jerked open, and the din is overwhelming.

Pushing through the crowd to you is the student body director. "We've got a real mess in there. The folding bleachers have partially collapsed on the north side of the gym. It is our homecoming game, and the place was packed. I saw a lot of blood, and kids are screaming for help."

Your first course of action should be

1. to triage all the victims
2. to set up a treatment center
3. to complete a size-up
4. to notify the nearest hospital

In the fire service the term "size up" refers to a rapid evaluation of the emergency made by the first-in officer in charge. Within moments he or she must consider a score of facts, resources, possible courses of action, and anticipated probable results that will affect the ability to bring an incident under control. As an initial responder to a multiple casualty incident (MCI), you may be called upon to size up the scope of your emergency, a task that may at first seem overwhelming. You will want to quickly assess some or all of the following.

Type of incident. Simply describe what you see. For example, "We have a passenger train derailment with fire," or "We have a three-story building collapse with an unknown number of victims trapped." Be clear and concise.

Location. Give as precise a location as possible. Use cross streets, hundred blocks, major intersections, or landmarks to alert incoming personnel.

Life hazards. Determine if any immediate life hazards are present. Fire, toxic gases, hazardous materials, flooding, traffic, or imminent structural collapse may pose a serious threat to survivors and rescue personnel alike.

Number of victims. Attempt to estimate the number of victims involved. This will directly affect the amount of resource equipment and personnel requested. Common sense must influence your judgment. A commercial bus may carry 50 passengers, a fully loaded jetliner may have 150 to 250 passengers on board, a large explosion with fire in an apartment complex at 4:00 A.M. could claim an unknown number of victims.

Fire department vehicles are now beginning to arrive at the scene. As first arriving medical unit your job is to set up an organized medical command post to coordinate the rescue effort. Your partner requests two engine companies to begin the triage of victims inside.

Which of the following is the best criterion for triaging multiple patients:

1. body system involved (i.e., respiratory, CNS, circulatory)
2. presence or absence of obvious trauma
3. urgency and survival potential
4. immediate threat to ABCs

Simplicity in the triage system is paramount. Many EMS systems use categories based on threats to the ABCs similar to the following outline.

Immediate. This category is for life-threatening injuries that require minimal intervention to correct. The requirement for short, quick intervention limits this category to airway problems and isolated bleeding.

Delayed. For this category victims have sustained significant anatomic injuries that require treatment but do not pose an immediate threat to the ABCs.

Walking wounded. This category includes those victims with minimal injuries who are able to aid themselves and possibly help others.

Dead/dying. This category encompasses those victims beyond help or with treatment needs so extensive and their chances for survival so limited that they do not warrant attention until other victims have been processed or until more resources arrive.

The performing of triage should be delegated to an initial responder or team whose medical expertise will allow them to evaluate and place all victims quickly into one of these categories. Marking victims can be as sophisticated as a color-coded tag attached to hand or foot or as simple as a category number placed on each victim's forehead with a marking pen.

As your partner distributes triage tags to the triage teams, you quickly confer with the fire department incident commander. Your request for 15 additional ambulances is acknowledged, and arriving police units initiate crowd control.

Inside the gymnasium the triage team walks into a chaotic scene. At least 80 to 90 persons are injured, trapped, or dead. There is confusion and suffering everywhere. The area is quickly sectored off to avoid duplicating the sorting effort, and walking wounded victims are ordered to gather in an uninvolved corner of the building. Within 15 minutes the task is done. There are 28 "immediate" victims, 37 "delayed" victims, 45 "walking wounded" and 6 "dead."

As medical commander your next step will probably be to set up a

1. treatment center
2. staging area
3. triage area
4. news conference

Once triage is complete, patients must be moved to a central location within or near the disaster area. At the treatment center, organized teams of EMTs, paramedics, or hospital staff sent to the scene perform necessary basic emergency care. Advanced life support procedures are generally not performed except on a limited number of critical care patients and then only as availability of trained personnel permits.

From this point, patients are prepared for transport from the adjacent ambulance loading area. A landing zone for helicopters can be established in a nearby area that is unobstructed to approach and departure and distant enough from the treatment center to avoid excessive noise and blown debris.

Ambulances begin to arrive and you direct them to stage near the entrance to the school parking lot. By now news media have gathered at the scene and are requesting information from your command post. An effective way to handle members of the media at an MCI is to

1. refuse to give information to any of them until initial rescue efforts are terminated
2. restrict media to the staging area, but keep them informed

3. request that each agency send only one representative into the disaster area
4. permit all authorized media representatives into the disaster area

News media may be permitted into the staging area as approved by the incident commander but should be kept out of the actual disaster area until a safe and secured status has been declared. In addition, a public information officer should be appointed to release approved bulletins to the press.

Your partner returns to your location to check on progress of the incident. Radio traffic to your command post is heavy and somewhat confusing. Your partner coordinates communication with the area hospital directing patient destinations as ambulances are being loaded with the first victims to be transported. Despite the chaotic scene before you, your organization is functioning reasonably well. In just over an hour all the "immediate" and 'delayed" victims have been taken to six different hospitals. "Walking wounded" are next and receive first aid treatment at the scene. The incident commander ensures the safeguarding of the fatalities until proper disposition can be made by the coroner or medical examiner.

An investigation by authorities later concludes that overloading and design failure led to the tragic collapse of the folding bleacher.

Discussion

Few may ever respond to a large-scale MCI apart from mockups and drills. A plan to deal with such a disaster, however, is mandatory for any progressive EMS system and allied agencies. While formulation may be at the bureaucratic level, the final result must be a simple workable guideline that is easily understood and implemented. Terminology will probably vary from plan to plan, but it is negligent not to be prepared. Your role as an initial responder may also be varied. Proper communications, flexibility, a central command, and a preestablished emergency disaster plan may well help avoid a "disastrous" response.

RELATED ASSESSMENT QUESTIONS

15.1 If you are having trouble transmitting over your radio, you might consider augmenting your antenna. Which of the following maneuvers would be least likely to improve your transmitting capabilities:
(a) switch to a high-gain antenna
(b) reposition the antenna to avoid close obstacles
(c) attach the antenna to a large metal object

(d) unplug other radios that might be on in the room
(e) begin transport and reattempt communication as your geographic position changes

15.2 Which of the following is *least* likely to be included in your initial radio report to the hospital:
(a) overview of the scene
(b) chief complaint
(c) severity
(d) level of consciousness
(e) current medications

15.3 Which of the following is included in good radio reporting skills:
(a) speak clearly and concisely
(b) handle disagreements discretely
(c) notify the hospital of changes in patient condition
(d) use an organized format to report information
(e) all of the above

15.4 *Line-of-sight* communication means that
(a) you must be able to see the receiving station
(b) the radio signal is unidirectional
(c) the radio must be operated outdoors
(d) the signal travels short distances and is easily blocked
(e) the antenna must point directly at the hospital

15.5 *Duplex* operation refers to
(a) the combination of the paramedic radio and the hospital radio
(b) the capability of transmitting and receiving simultaneously
(c) a feature that records EKG while also transmitting it
(d) one paramedic acting as patient medic and the other as radio medic
(e) the use of the paramedic radio as a repeater

15.6 If the paramedic radio fails to function properly, you can check all of the following *except*
(a) battery condition
(b) proper channel selection
(c) signal strength
(d) antenna connection
(e) proper mode selection

15.7 Under certain conditions you may be able to receive the hospital's transmission loud and clear, but it is unable to copy yours. The *least* probable explanation for this is
(a) adverse weather conditions
(b) obstructive terrain between your radio and the hospital
(c) your private line function is "off"
(d) simultaneous radio traffic with another field unit
(e) internal malfunction of either radio

15.8 Paramedic telemetry radios operate in which of the following frequency ranges:
(a) AM
(b) FM
(c) VHF
(d) UHF
(e) SW

15.9 Information that you would probably not include in your initial report to the hospital on a patient with chest pain is
(a) patient's age
(b) patient's sex
(c) chief complaint
(d) level of consciousness
(e) allergies

15.10 An antenna must be used in order to
(a) transmit only
(b) receive only
(c) both transmit and receive
(d) adjust the squelch
(e) operate the radio except as a repeater

15.11 You and your partner are at the same scene of a traffic accident with the following patients. Which one will fall into the triage category to be left untreated unless more help arrives:
(a) 39-year-old male with chest trauma and difficulty breathing
(b) his 38-year-old wife, who is in full arrest from major abdominal injuries
(c) their 5-year-old child, who has a scalp laceration and is vomiting
(d) a 65-year-old man with facial injuries and stertorous breathing
(e) his 60-year-old wife, who has a fractured femur and multiple small lacerations about the face

ANSWER KEY

15.1 d	**15.4** d	**15.7** a	**15.10** c
15.2 e	**15.5** b	**15.8** d	**15.11** b
15.3 e	**15.6** c	**15.9** e	

INDEX

A

B

C

D

E

F

G

H

S

T

V

W